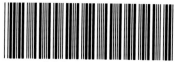

APOS CLINICAL REFERENCE HANDBOOKS

Psycho-Oncology: A Quick Reference on the Psychosocial Dimensions of Cancer Symptom Management, 2nd edition, Jimmie C. Holland, Mitch Golant, Donna B. Greenberg, Mary K. Hughes, Jon A. Levenson, Matthew J. Loscalzo, William F. Pirl

Pediatric Psycho-Oncology: A Quick Reference on the Psychosocial Dimensions of Cancer Symptom Management, 2nd edition, Lori S. Wiener, Maryland Pao, Anne E. Kazak, Mary Jo Kupst, Andrea Farkas Patenaude

Geriatric Psycho-Oncology: A Quick Reference on the Psychosocial Dimensions of Cancer Symptom Management, Jimmie C. Holland, Talia Weiss Wiesel, Christian J. Nelson, Andrew J. Roth, Yesne Alici

Contents

Foreword

Geriatric oncology is a rapidly evolving field of medicine. The overall increase in life expectancy results in rapidly changing demographics with significant aging of the world population. As cancer incidence and cancer mortality increase with age, the number of older adults with cancer will represent a significant challenge in the future of public health.

Older adults have very special needs. As a geriatrician taking care of patients in a comprehensive cancer center, I am constantly surprised by the complexity of the medical care of patients who, in addition to their cancer diagnosis, have an incredibly high prevalence of frailty, multiplicity of disease, disabilities, and decline in their functional reserve, cognitive impairment, and progressive restriction in personal and social resources. The distress associated with surgery, radiation, chemotherapy, pain, and other symptoms related to cancer and cancer treatment is complicated by psychiatric and psychological issues found more frequently in the aging patient, such as undiagnosed mental illness, memory impairment and loneliness, lack of social support, or caregiver stress.

Oncologists may not be aware of the geriatric-specific issues that need to be addressed in addition to usual care. Are they communicating well with the patient? Is the patient understanding the important nuances of the treatment decisions? Are they obtaining consent correctly? Are the family members interfering with or dictating patient's wishes? Who will provide advance directives?

This Handbook is written for oncologists, nurses, and other health professionals who are treating older adults and are often unfamiliar with the diagnosis and management of psychiatric comorbidities in cancer. The authors address psychiatric disorders and psychosocial issues specific to symptoms and cancer sites. In addition, several chapters cover unique problems of the elderly such as communication, social isolation, and issues related to elderly care in minority groups. The final section describes possible interventions and available resources for elderly cancer patients.

This Handbook stresses practical aspects of care and provides guidelines for the clinicians as they strive to understand and manage the psychiatric and psychological aspects of the disease. It will be invaluable in providing a rapid and comprehensive source of information about criteria for diagnosis and medications with dosages and precautions. Older patient's care will be enhanced by the fact that it will be easier for oncologists to deliver "whole patient" care that pays proper attention to the emotional as well as the physical aspects. The Handbook authors are largely from Memorial Sloan Kettering Cancer Center's Geriatric Psychiatry and 65+ Hospital Program.

However, there are valued contributors from several other centers. It is the hope that the Handbook will help oncologists in their care of elders with cancer in their practice.

Beatriz Korc-Grodzicki, MD, PhD
Chief, Geriatrics Service
Department of Medicine
Memorial Sloan Kettering Cancer Center
New York, New York

Preface

This book joins APOS Clinical Reference Handbooks Series developed to provide a rapid pocket-sized "curbside consultation" for busy oncologic physicians and their teams on the common psychiatric and psychological problems confronted by children with cancer, adults—and now this edition for older adults. The crisis in care of elders in our society is evolving rapidly because of an unusual confluence of factors: the swell of the elder population by the baby boomer generation's reaching 65 and the fact that we are living longer as elders with more comorbidities which require chronic medical care. These factors impact upon cancer care particularly, which is now the leading cause of death, since heart disease is now better prevented and treated and moves down to the second leading cause of death. Importantly as well, is the fact that the medical care system has not produced the number of much needed and hoped for geriatricians with expertise to care for this burgeoning population. Nor have we increased the numbers of geriatric psychiatrists to act as consultants to the physicians providing medical care to elders. Thus, this handbook fills a need to assure that physicians caring for elders have ready access to information about the most commonly encountered problems: anxiety and how to treat it without sedation; depression and deciding the cause and best treatment; recognizing poor judgment and assessing for early cognitive problems; supporting elders in the face of ageism in society, which is easily transmitted to medical teams who become impatient with the slower and more difficult communication. Fatigue, pain, and sexual dysfunction, often overlooked and neglected, are discussed. This handbook also reviews the problems common to particular sites of cancer in elders: breast, prostate, colon, lung, and lymphoma. What are the safest pharmacologic interventions and precautions? What psychosocial (nonpharmacologic) interventions have been tried and are effective with elders? All are reviewed in chapters that deal with each.

The quality of medical care has improved in the last decade in part due to the development of guidelines and checklists to assure full assessment. This has been highly evident in oncologic care of elders who, for so long, were excluded from cancer treatments based on age alone. A chapter by Wildes deals with rapid clinical functional assessment that recognizes that age alone is not a measure of appropriateness for chemotherapy or surgery but, rather, how the person is functioning in all areas of physical, social, psychological domains. Similarly, the use of scales to rapidly measure cognitive function and the presence of depression or anxiety has proven to be helpful to clinicians who are busy in clinics where time is a factor. The handbook presents these and also suggests referral to the *NCCN Guidelines for Senior Adults* and the *Distress Management Guidelines,* which outline issues in the broader aspects of adult cancer care.

Jimmie C. Holland, MD
Wayne E. Chapman
Chair in Psychiatric Oncology
Attending Psychiatrist
Department of Psychiatry & Behavioral Sciences
Memorial Sloan Kettering Cancer Center
New York, New York
January 2014

Contributors

Tim A. Ahles, PhD
Director
Neurocognitive
Research Laboratory
Department of Psychiatry &
Behavioral Sciences
Memorial Sloan Kettering Cancer
Center
Professor of Psychology in
Psychiatry
Department of Psychiatry
Weill Cornell Medical College
New York, New York

Yesne Alici, MD
Assistant Attending Psychiatrist
Memorial Sloan Kettering Cancer
Center
Assistant Professor of Psychiatry
Weill Medical College of Cornell
University
New York, New York

Charissa Andreotti, PhD
Department of Psychiatry &
Behavioral Sciences
Memorial Sloan Kettering Cancer
Center
New York, New York

Lea Baider, PhD
Professor of Medical Psychology
Hebrew University Medical School
Department of Psychiatry
Sharett Institute of Oncology
Hadassah Medical Center
Jerusalem, Israel

John W. Barnhill, MD
Attending Psychiatrist
New York-Presbyterian Hospital
Professor of Clinical Psychiatry
and Public Health
Weill Cornell Medical College
New York, New York

Archana Bushan, MD
Fellow, Hospice and Palliative
Medicine
Department of Medicine
Memorial Sloan Kettering Cancer
Center
New York, New York

Matthew N. Doolittle, MD
Department of Psychiatry &
Behavioral Sciences
Memorial Sloan Kettering Cancer
Center
New York, New York

Daisuke Fujisawa, MD, PhD
Center for Psychiatric Oncology
and Behavioral Sciences
Massachusetts General Hospital
Boston, Massachusetts

**Barbara A. Given, PhD,
RN, FAAN**
Director of PhD Program
College of Nursing
Michigan State University
East Lansing, Michigan

Mindy Greenstein, PhD
Clinical Psychologist
New York, New York

Elizabeth Harvey, PhD
Department of Psychiatry &
Behavioral Sciences
Memorial Sloan Kettering Cancer
Center
New York, New York

Jimmie C. Holland, MD
Wayne E. Chapman Chair in
Psychiatric Oncology
Department of Psychiatry &
Behavioral Sciences
Memorial Sloan Kettering Cancer
Center
New York, New York

**Mary K. Hughes, MS, RN,
CNS, CT**
Clinical Nurse Specialist
Department of Psychiatry
The University of Texas MD
Anderson Cancer Center
Houston, Texas

R. Garrett Key, MD
Department of Psychiatry &
Behavioral Sciences
Memorial Sloan Kettering Cancer
Center
New York, New York

Kenneth L. Kirsh, PhD
Clinical Research Educator
and Research Scientist
Millennium Research Institute
San Diego, California

Stephanie Lacey, MA, LMHC
Research Project Coordinator
Department of Psychiatry &
Behavioral Sciences
Memorial Sloan Kettering Cancer
Center
New York, New York

Tomer T. Levin, MBBS, FAPM
Department of Psychiatry &
Behavioral Sciences
Memorial Sloan Kettering Cancer
Center
New York, New York

Anne Martin, PhD, LCSW
Clinical Supervisor/Program
Manager
Social Work Services
Memorial Sloan Kettering Cancer
Center
New York, New York

Mary Jane Massie, MD
Department of Psychiatry &
Behavioral Sciences
Memorial Sloan Kettering Cancer
Center
New York, New York

Kimberley Miller, MD, FRCPC
Attending Psychiatrist
Department of Psychosocial
Oncology and Palliative Care
Princess Margaret Cancer Centre
Assistant Professor
University of Toronto
Toronto, Canada

Nicholas Miller
Millennium Research Institute
San Diego, California

Christian J. Nelson, PhD
Clinical Psychologist
Department of Psychiatry &
Behavioral Sciences
Memorial Sloan Kettering Cancer
Center
Assistant Professor of Psychology
Weill Cornell Medical College
New York, New York

Steven D. Passik, PhD
Director of Clinical Addiction
Research and Education
Millennium Laboratories
San Diego, California

William F. Pirl, MD, MPH

Associate Professor of Psychiatry
Harvard Medical School
Director, Center for Psychiatric
Oncology and Behavioral
Sciences
Massachusetts General Hospital
Boston, Massachusetts

James C. Root, PhD

Department of Psychiatry &
Behavioral Sciences
Memorial Sloan Kettering Cancer
Center
Assistant Professor of Psychology
Departments of Psychiatry and
Anesthesiology
Weill Cornell Medical College
New York, New York

Andrew J. Roth, MD

Psychiatrist
Department of Psychiatry &
Behavioral Sciences
Memorial Sloan Kettering Cancer
Center
Professor of Clinical Psychiatry
Weill Cornell Medical College
New York, New York

Matthew Ruehle

Millennium Research Institute
San Diego, California

Adam Rzetelny, PhD

Millennium Research Institute
San Diego, California

Steven Schulberg, BA

Department of Psychiatry &
Behavioral Sciences
Memorial Sloan Kettering Cancer
Center
New York, New York

Tatiana D. Starr, MA

Clinical Research Coordinator
Department of Psychiatry &
Behavioral Sciences
Memorial Sloan Kettering Cancer
Center
New York, New York

Roma Tickoo, MD, MPH

Assistant Attending
Palliative Medicine Service
Department of Medicine
Memorial Sloan Kettering Cancer
Center
New York, New York

**Mark I. Weinberger,
PhD, MPH**

Vice President of Clinical Services
and Associate Director of
Clinical Research
The IMA Group
Clinical Instructor of Psychology in
Psychiatry
Weill Cornell Medical College
New York, New York

Talia Weiss Wiesel, PhD

Psychology Intern
New York Presbyterian Hospital/
Weill Cornell Medical College
Department of Psychiatry &
Behavioral Sciences
Memorial Sloan Kettering Cancer
Center
New York, New York

Tanya M. Wildes, MD, MSCI

Assistant Professor of Medicine
Division of Medical Oncology
Washington University School of
Medicine
St. Louis, Missouri

Section I

Screening and Interventions

Chapter 1

Psychosocial Screening Instruments for Older Cancer Patients

William F. Pirl, Stephanie Lacey, and Mark I. Weinberger

Introduction

Many instruments have been developed to assess psychosocial distress and its subtypes in geriatric cancer patients. Although the clinician may not employ them often in clinical care, they do help in identifying the presence and severity of a particular symptom. This chapter provides a guide to these instruments. The chapter is organized according to the NCCN Distress algorithm, starting with a single-item tool to rapidly assess general psychosocial distress in the waiting room (i.e., the distress thermometer) followed by focusing on more specific areas of distress as the clinical evaluation proceeds.

General Distress

Distress Thermometer

The distress thermometer (Figure 1.1) is a 0–10 scale that asks patients to rate their distress.[1] Scores of 4 or above warrant further evaluation. The tool also contains a list of possible problems that patients can endorse to guide the clinician's evaluation of the distress and its appropriate treatment. These problems include practical, family, emotional, spiritual/religious, and physical problems. If a patient endorses yes on an item under Emotional Problems, clinicians could consider administering the Geriatric Depression Scale—Short Form (GDS—SF) and/or the Hospital Anxiety and Depression Scale (HADS). If a patient endorses yes on an item under Spiritual/Religious Concerns, clinicians might consider evaluating this further with the FICA Spiritual History Tool©. If a patient endorses yes to problems with memory/concentration under Physical Problems, consider further assessment with the Mini Mental Status Examination (MMSE) or the Blessed Orientation-Memory-Concentration Test (BOMC). See Figure 1.1.

Some forms of distress may not be readily identified by the distress thermometer such as substance abuse, dementia, and delirium. Based on

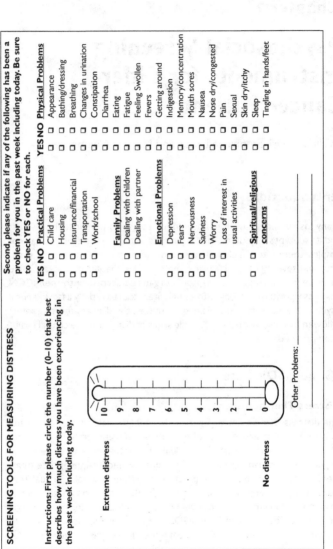

SCREENING TOOLS FOR MEASURING DISTRESS

Instructions: First please circle the number (0–10) that best describes how much distress you have been experiencing in the past week including today.

Extreme distress

10
9
8
7
6
5
4
3
2
1
0

No distress

Other Problems: _____

Second, please indicate if any of the following has been a problem for you in the past week including today. Be sure to check YES or NO for each.

YES	NO	Practical Problems	YES	NO	Physical Problems
☐	☐	Child care	☐	☐	Appearance
☐	☐	Housing	☐	☐	Bathing/dressing
☐	☐	Insurance/financial	☐	☐	Breathing
☐	☐	Transportation	☐	☐	Changes in urination
☐	☐	Work/school	☐	☐	Constipation
			☐	☐	Diarrhea
		Family Problems	☐	☐	Eating
☐	☐	Dealing with children	☐	☐	Fatigue
☐	☐	Dealing with partner	☐	☐	Feeling Swollen
			☐	☐	Fevers
		Emotional Problems	☐	☐	Getting around
☐	☐	Depression	☐	☐	Indigestion
☐	☐	Fears	☐	☐	Memory/concentration
☐	☐	Nervousness	☐	☐	Mouth sores
☐	☐	Sadness	☐	☐	Nausea
☐	☐	Worry	☐	☐	Nose dry/congested
☐	☐	Loss of interest in usual activities	☐	☐	Pain
			☐	☐	Sexual
		Spiritual/religious concerns	☐	☐	Skin dry/itchy
☐	☐		☐	☐	Sleep
			☐	☐	Tingling in hands/feet

Figure 1.1 NCCN Distress Management Guideline DIS-A—Distress Thermometer. Adapted from *Screening Tools for Measuring Distress* [CD-Rom]. Jenkintown, PA: National Comprehensive Cancer Network; May 2005.

the patient's history and clinical presentation, other assessments should be done for further evaluation. For substance abuse, consider the Short Michigan Alcoholism Screening Instrument—Geriatric Version (SMAST-G) and the CAGE (acronym for Cut down, Annoyed, Guilty, Eye-opener) questionnaire described under Substance Abuse in this chapter. If there is concern about possible dementia, tests such as the MMSE and the Clock Drawing Test should be considered. If there is concern about delirium, the Memorial Delirium Assessment Scale (MDAS) should be considered. Concerns about dementia and delirium are explained further under Cognition in this chapter.

Emotional Problems

Geriatric Depression Scale—Short Form (GDS—SF)

Depression is one of the most common causes of emotional distress in the elderly and continues to be under-recognized.[2,3,4] Unfortunately, depression can have deleterious effects on quality of life and depressive symptoms are linked to poor health outcomes and increasing costs of health care.[4,5] Furthermore, depression is one of the top five concerns of the elderly.[4] The Geriatric Depression Scale—Short Form (GDS-SF) (Table 1.1) is a self-report measure of depression in older adults featuring an uncomplicated yes/no response format. Although originally developed as a 30-item instrument, a 15-item version (GDS-SF) was formed to decrease the length of time it takes to complete.

Hospital Anxiety and Depression Scale

As opposed to the GDS-SF, which solely measures depression, the Hospital Anxiety and Depression Scale (HADS) (Figure 1.2) is a 14-item self-report instrument that assesses both anxiety and depressive symptoms (seven items assess anxiety and seven items assess depression).[6] The instrument was designed for medically ill patients and does not include physical symptoms. A total score is derived from all 14 items with subscales for anxiety and depression. It has been validated in patients with cancer and may be the most widely used instrument to assess depressive symptoms in cancer patients. Scores on the HADS do not diagnose anxiety and mood disorders; they measure the severity of symptoms that suggest the likeliness that a patient may have a disorder. A total score of 15 or greater or a score of 8 or greater on a subscale suggests that a patient may have an anxiety or mood disorder. However, in psychosocial research, the cut-off scores for the HADS can vary and some believe that higher scores are necessary to increase the specificity of the instrument. The HADS testing materials can be purchased directly from GL Assessment (www.gl-assessment.co.uk).

Table 1.1 Geriatric Depression Scale—Short Form (GDS—SF)		
Please circle the most appropriate response:		
1) Are you basically satisfied with your life?	Yes	No
2) Have you dropped many of your activities and interests?	Yes	No
3) Do you feel your life is empty?	Yes	No
4) Do you often get bored?	Yes	No
5) Are you in good spirits most of the time?	Yes	No
6) Are you afraid that something bad is going to happen to you?	Yes	No
7) Do you feel happy most of the time?	Yes	No
8) Do you often feel helpless?	Yes	No
9) Do you prefer to stay at home rather than go out and do new things?	Yes	No
10) Do you feel that you have more problems with memory than most?	Yes	No
11) Do you think it is wonderful to be alive now?	Yes	No
12) Do you feel pretty worthless the way you are now?	Yes	No
13) Do you feel full of energy?	Yes	No
14) Do you feel your situation is hopeless?	Yes	No
15) Do you think most people are better off than you?	Yes	No

Adapted from Sheikh JI YJ. Geriatric Depression Scale (GDS): recent evidence and development of a shorter version. *J Clin Gerontol & Geriatr.* 1986;5(1/2):165–173.

Cognition

Mini Mental Status Examination

The Mini Mental Status Examination (MMSE) (Figure 1.3) is a 14-item clinician-administered instrument to assess cognition, regardless of cause.[7] It contains items on orientation, attention, recall, visual-spatial construction, and language abilities. Scores of 24 or less suggest severe impairment. Further neuropsychological assessment is often needed for dementia, particularly with assessments that include tests of frontal lobe functioning. The MMSE can be used serially to follow patients at risk for developing cognitive impairment or patients who have had alterations in their cognition, particularly by delirium. MMSE testing materials can be purchased directly from PAR, Inc. (www.parinc.com).

Blessed Orientation-Memory-Concentration Test (BOMC)

If a shorter assessment is preferred, the BOMC (Table 1.2) is a 6-question test that screens for gross cognitive impairment and discriminates between patients with mild, moderate, and severe cognitive deficits.[8] This assessment tests orientation, recall, and attention with scores between 10 and

HADS

Please read each item and CIRCLE the answer that comes closest to how you have been feeling, on the average, IN THE PAST WEEK. Don't spend too much time on your answers: Your immediate reaction to each item will probably be more accurate than a long thought-out response.

1. I feel tense or "wound up":
   a. Most of the time
   b. A lot of the time
   c. From time to time
   d. Not at all

2. I still enjoy the things I used to enjoy:
   a. Definitely as much
   b. Not quite so much
   c. Only a little
   d. Hardly at all

3. I get a sort of frightened feeling as if something awful is about to happen:
   a. Very definitely and quite badly
   b. Yes, but not too badly
   c. A little, but it doesn't worry me
   d. Not at all

4. I can laugh and see the funny side of things:
   a. As much as I always could
   b. Not quite so much now
   c. Definitely not so much now
   d. Not at all

5. Worrying thoughts go through my mind:
   a. A great deal of the time
   b. A lot of the time
   c. From time too time but not too often
   d. Only occasionally

6. I feel cheerful:
   a. Not at all
   b. Not often
   c. Sometimes
   d. Most of the time

7. I can sit at ease and feel relaxed:
   a. Definitely
   b. Usually
   c. Not often
   d. Not at all

8. I feel as if I am slowed down:
   a. Nearly all the time
   b. Very often
   c. Sometimes
   d. Not at all

9. I get a sort of frightened feeling like "butterflies" in my stomach:
   a. Not at all
   b. Occasionally
   c. Quite often
   d. Very often

10. I have lost interest in my appearance:
    a. Definitely
    b. I don't take as much care as I should
    c. I may not take quite as much care
    d. I take just as much care as ever

11. I feel restless as if I have to be on the move:
    a. Very much indeed
    b. Quite a lot
    c. Not very much
    d. Not at all

12. I look forward with enjoyment to things:
    a. As much as I ever did
    b. Rather less than I used to
    c. Definitely less than I used to
    d. Hardly at all

13. I get sudden feelings of panic:
    a. Very often indeed
    b. Quite often
    c. Not very often
    d. Not at all

14. I can enjoy a good book or radio or TV program:
    a. Often
    b. Sometimes
    c. Not often
    d. Very seldom

Figure 1.2 Hospital Anxiety and Depression Scale (HADS). Adapted from Zigmond AS, Snaith RP. The hospital anxiety and depression scale. *Acta psychiatrica Scandinavica.* Jun 1983;67(6):361–370.

INSTRUCTIONS FOR ADMINISTRATION OF MINI MENTAL STATUS EXAMINATION

ORIENTATION

1. Ask for the date. Then ask specifically for parts omitted.
   i.e., "Can you also tell me what season it is?" One point for each correct.
2. Ask in turn, "Can you tell me the name of this place?", town, county, etc. One point for each correct.

REGISTRATION

Tell the person you are going to test their memory. Then say the names of three unrelated objects, clearly and slowly, about one second for each. After you have said all three, ask him to repeat them. This first repetition determines his score (0–3) but keep saying them until he can repeat all three, up to six trials. If the subject does not eventually learn all three, recall cannot be meaningfully tested.

ATTENTION AND CALCULATION

Ask the subject to begin with 100 and count backwards by 7. Stop after five subtractions. Score the total number of correct answers.

If the subject cannot or will not perform this task, ask him to spell the word "world" backwards. The score is the number of letters in correct order.
   i.e., dlrow = 5 points, dlorw = 3 points.

RECALL

Ask the patient if he can recall the three words you previously asked him to remember. One point for each correctly recalled.

LANGUAGE

Naming: Show the subject a wristwatch and ask her what it is.

Repeat with a pencil. One point for each named correctly.

Repetition: Ask the patient to repeat the sentence after you. Allow only one trial.

3 Stage Command: give the verbal instructions, then present the subject a sheet of paper. One point for each part of the command that is correctly executed.

Reading: Have the subject read the phrase "CLOSE YOUR EYES". The letters should be large and dark enough for the subject to read. Ask him to "Read the sentence and do what it says." Score correctly only if they read the phrase and close their eyes.

Writing: Give the subject a blank piece of paper and ask her write a sentence for you. Do not dictate a sentence, it is to be written by the subject spontaneously. To score correctly, it must contain a subject and verb and be sensible. It should be a complete thought. Correct grammar and punctuation are NOT necessary.

Copying: On a piece of paper, draw intersecting pentagons, each side about one inch and ask him to copy it exactly as it is. To score correctly, all ten angles must be present AND two must intersect. Tremor and rotation are ignored.

Estimate the subject's level of sensorium along a continuum, from alert to coma.

TOTAL SCORE POSSIBLE = 30
23 OR LESS: HIGH LIKELIHOOD OF DEMENTIA
25–30: NORMAL AGING OR BORDERLINE DEMENTIA

Figure 1.3 Mini Mental Status Examination (MMSE). Adapted from Folstein MF, Folstein SE, McHugh PR. "Mini-mental state". a practical method for grading the cognitive state of patients for the clinician. *J Psychiatr Res*. Nov 1975;12(3):189–198.

MINI MENTAL STATUS EXAM

PATEINT'S NAME: _____

Date: _____   Client's Highest Level of Education: _____

Maximum Score	Score	ORIENTATION
5	( )	What is the (year) (season) (date) (day) (month)?
5	( )	where are we: (state) (county) (town) (hospital (floor)?

REGISTRATION

3	( )	Name 3 objects: One syllable words, 1 second to say each.
		Then ask the patient all 3 after you have said them.
		Give 1 point for each correct answer. Then repeat them until he learns all 3.
		Count trials and record. Trials _____

ATTENTION AND CALCULATION

5	( )	Serial 7's. 1 point for each correct. Stop after 5 answers. Alternatively spell "world" backwards.
		100 – 93 – 86 – 79 – 72 – 65 – 58

RECALL

3	( )	Ask for 3 objects repeated above. Give 1 point for each correct.

LANGUAGE

9	( )	Name a pencil, and watch (2 points)
	( )	Repeat the following: "No ifs, and or buts." (1 point)
	( )	Follow a 3-stage command: "Take this paper in your right hand, fold it in half, and put it on the floor." (3 points)
	( )	Read and obey the following: "Close your eyes" (1 point)
	( )	Write a sentence. (1 point)
	( )	Copy design. (1 point)

_____
Total Score

Assess level of consciousness _____
along a continuum.   (Alert)   (Drowsy)   (Stupor)   (Coma)

Figure 1.3 (Continued)

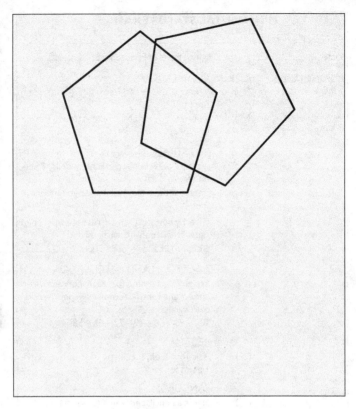

Close your eyes.

Figure 1.3 (Continued)

28 suggesting symptoms related to dementia or cognitive impairment. For scores between 0 and 9 when patients are exhibiting cognitive symptoms, further assessments are recommended, such as the MMSE.

Clock Drawing Test

The Clock Drawing Test (Figure 1.4) is a pen-and-paper test that assesses several cognitive abilities. It is a good adjuvant test of executive functioning when given with the MMSE (Figure 1.3).[9] Patients are asked to draw a clock on a piece of paper, putting the numbers on the face, and making the hands on the clock designate a specific time, such as ten minutes before two. This task tests patients' ability to follow complex commands and sequence and plan their actions, as well as their visual-spatial ability. The drawn clock can be objectively scored by a validated scoring system. There are two scoring

Table 1.2 The Blessed-Orientation-Memory-Concentration

Test Score of 1 for each incorrect response: Maximum weighted error score = 28

Questions	Maximal Error	X	Score	=	Weight
1. What year is it now?	1	X	4	=	
2. What month is it now?	1	X	3	=	
3. Memory Phrase: Repeat this phrase after me: *John Brown* *42 Market Street, Chicago*		X		=	
4. About what time is it? (Within 1 hour)	1	X	3	=	
5. Count backwards 20–1	1 or 2	X	2	=	
6. Say the months in reverse order	1 or 2	X	2	=	
7. Repeat the Memory Phrase: John (1); Brown (2); 42 (3) Market Street (4); Chicago (5)	1,2,3,4 or 5	X	2	=	
TOTAL =					

Adapted from Katzman R, Brown T, Fuld P, Peck A, Schechter R, Schimmel H. Validation of a short Orientation-Memory-Concentration Test of cognitive impairment. *Am J Psychiat.* Jun 1983;140(6):734–739.

systems, each of which has reasonable sensitivity and specificity in identifying cognitive dysfunction.[10,11] In the Sunderland et al. method, scores of 6 or more are considered normal.[11]

Memorial Delirium Assessment Scale

The Memorial Delirium Assessment Scale (MDAS; Box 1.1) is a 10-item clinician-administered assessment that evaluates the areas of cognition most sensitive to impairment with delirium: arousal, level of consciousness, memory, attention, orientation, disturbances in thinking, and psychomotor activity.[12] Scores range from 0 to 30, and scores of 13 or more suggests delirium. This scale, when used serially, monitors changes in function.

Substance Abuse

Short Michigan Alcoholism Screening Instrument—Geriatric Version

The Short Michigan Alcoholism Screening Instrument—Geriatric version (SMAST-G; (Box 1.2) is a 10-item questionnaire in yes/no format that is used to identify older adults who are at risk for an alcohol disorder (i.e., abuse or dependence). A score of two or more (each yes endorsement equals one point) suggests alcohol abuse and warrants

Please draw the numbers on the circle to make it look like a clock. Then please draw the hands of the clock to read <u>10 past 11</u>.

<u>Watson et al Scoring Method:</u>
1. Divide the circle into 4 equal quadrants by drawing one line through the center of the circle and the number 12 (or a mark that best corresponds to the 12) and a second line perpendicular to and bisecting the first.
2. Count the number of digits in each quadrant in the clockwise direction, beginning with the digit corresponding to the number 12. Each digit is counted only once. If a digit falls on one of the reference lines, it is included in the quadrant that is clockwise to the line. A total of 3 digits in a quadrant is considered to be correct.
3. For any error in the number of digits in the first, second or third quadrants assign a score of 1. For any error in the number of digits in the fourth quadrant assign a score of 4.
4. Normal range of score is 0-3. Abnormal (demented) range of score is 4-7.

<u>Sunderland et al Scoring Method:</u>
Score
10-6 **Drawing of clock face with circle and number is generally intact.**
10   Hands are in correct position.
9   Slight errors in placement of the hands.
8   More noticeable errors in the placement of hour and minute hands.
7   Placement of hands is significantly off course.
6   Inappropriate use of clock hands (i.e. use of digital display or circling of numbers despite repeated instructions).
5-1 **Drawing of clock face with circle and numbers is *not* intact.**
5   Crowding of numbers at one end of the clock or reversal of numbers. Hands may still be present in some fashion.
4   Further distortion of number sequence. Integrity of clock face is now gone (i.e. numbers missing or placed at outside of the boundaries of the clock face).
3   Numbers and clock face no longer obviously connected in the drawing. Hands are not present.
2   Drawing reveals some evidence of instructions being received but only a vague representation of a clock.
1   Either no attempt or an uninterpretable effort is made.

Figure 1.4 Clock Drawing Test. Adapted from Sunderland T, Hill JL, Mellow AM, et al. Clock drawing in Alzheimer's disease. A novel measure of dementia severity. *J Am Geriatr Soc.* Aug 1989;37(8):725–729.

additional assessment and potential interventions.[13] The SMAST-G can be used to identify patients whose drinking patterns increase their probability for various health problems such as liver disease, heart disease, or stroke.

Box 1.1 Memorial Delirium Assessment Scale

Instructions: Rate the severity of the following symptoms of delirium based on current interaction with subject or assessment of his/her behavior or experience over past several hours (as indicated in each time).

ITEM 1—REDUCED LEVEL OF CONSCIOUSNESS (AWARENESS): Rate the patient's current awareness of and interaction with the environment (interviewer, other people/objects in the room; for example, ask patients to describe their surroundings).

☐ 0: none (patient spontaneously fully aware of environment and interacts appropriately)

☐ 1: mild (patient is unaware of some elements in the environment or is not spontaneously interacting appropriately with the interviewer; becomes fully aware and appropriately interactive when prodded strongly; interview is prolonged but not seriously disrupted)

☐ 2: moderate (patient is unaware of some or all elements in the environment or is not spontaneously interacting with the interviewer; becomes incompletely aware and inappropriately interactive when prodded strongly; interview is prolonged but not seriously disrupted)

☐ 3: severe (patient is unaware of all elements in the environment with no spontaneous interaction or awareness of the interviewer so that the interview is difficult to impossible, even with maximal prodding)

ITEM 2—DISORIENTATION: Rate current state by asking the following 10 orientation items: date, month, day, year, season, floor, name of hospital, city, state, and country.

☐ 0: none (patient knows 9–10 items)

☐ 1: mild (patient knows 7–8 items)

☐ 2: moderate (patient knows 5–6 items)

☐ 3: severe (patient knows no more than 4 items)

ITEM 3—SHORT-TERM MEMORY IMPAIRMENT: Rate current state by using repetition and delayed recall of 3 words [patient must immediately repeat and recall words 5 minutes later after an intervening task. Use alternate sets of 3 words for successive evaluations (e.g., apple, table, tomorrow; sky, cigar, justice)].

☐ 0: none (all 3 words repeated and recalled)

☐ 1: mild (all 3 repeated; patient fails to recall 1)

☐ 2: moderate (all 3 repeated; patient fails to recall 2-3)

☐ 3: severe (patient fails to repeat 1 or more words)

ITEM 4—IMPAIRED DIGIT SPAN: Rate current performance by asking subjects to repeat first 3, 4, then 5 digits forward and then 3, then 4 backward; continue to the next step only if patient succeeds at the previous one.

☐ 0: none (patient can do at least 5 numbers forward, 4 backward)

☐ 1: mild (patient can do at least 5 numbers forward, 3 backward)

(continued)

Box 1.1 (Continued)

☐ 2: moderate (patient can do 4-5 numbers forward, cannot do 3 backward)

☐ 3: severe (patient can do no more than 3 numbers forward)

ITEM 5—REDUCED ABILITY TO MAINTAIN AND SHIFT ATTENTION: As indicated during the interview by questions needing to be rephrased and/or repeated because patient's attention wanders, patient loses track, patient is distracted by outside stimuli or overabsorbed in task.

☐ 0: none (none of the previously mentioned; patient maintains and shifts attention normally)

☐ 1: mild (previously mentioned attentional problems occur once or twice without prolonging the interview)

☐ 2: moderate (previously mentioned attentional problems occur often, prolonging the interview without seriously disrupting it)

☐ 3: severe (previously mentioned attentional problems occur constantly, disrupting and making the interview difficult to impossible)

ITEM 6—DISORGANIZED THINKING: As indicated during the interview by rambling, irrelevant, or incoherent speech, or by tangential, circumstantial, or faulty reasoning. Ask patient a somewhat complex question (e.g., "Describe your current medical condition.").

☐ 0: none (patient's speech is coherent and goal-directed)

☐ 1: mild (patient's speech is slightly difficult to follow; responses to questions are slightly off target but not so much as to prolong the interview)

☐ 2: moderate (disorganized thoughts or speech are clearly present, such that interview is prolonged but not disrupted)

☐ 3: severe (examination is very difficult or impossible due to disorganized thinking or speech)

ITEM 7—PERCEPTUAL DISTURBANCE: Misperceptions, illusions, hallucinations inferred from inappropriate behavior during the interview or admitted by the subject, as well as those elicited from nurse/family/chart accounts of the past several hours or of the time since last examination:

☐ 0: none (no misperceptions, illusions, or hallucinations)

☐ 1: mild (misperceptions or illusions related to sleep, fleeting hallucinations on 1-2 occasions without inappropriate behavior)

☐ 2: moderate (hallucinations or frequent illusions on several occasions with minimal inappropriate behavior that does not disrupt the interview)

☐ 3: severe (frequent or intense illusions or hallucinations with persistent inappropriate behavior that disrupts the interview or interferes with medical care)

(continued)

Box 1.1 (Continued)

ITEM 8—DELUSIONS: Rate delusions inferred from inappropriate behavior exhibited during the interview or admitted by the patient, as well as delusions elicited from nurse/family/chart accounts of the past several hours or of the time since the previous examination.

☐ 0: none (no evidence of misinterpretations or delusions)

☐ 1: mild (misinterpretation or suspiciousness without clear delusional ideas or inappropriate behavior)

☐ 2: moderate (delusions admitted by the patient or evidenced by his/her behavior that do not or only marginally disrupt the interview or interfere with medical care)

☐ 3: severe (persistent and/or intense delusions resulting in inappropriate behavior, disrupting the interview or seriously interfering with medical care)

ITEM 9—DECREASED OR INCREASED PSYCHOMOTOR ACTIVITY: Rate activity over past several hours, as well as activity during interview, by circling (a) hypoactive, (b) hyperactive, or (c) elements of both present.

☐ 0: none (normal psychomotor activity)

a b c ☐ 1: mild (Hypoactivity is barely noticeable, expressed as slightly slowing movement. Hyperactivity is barely noticeable or appears as simple restlessness.)

a b c ☐ 2: moderate (Hypoactivity is undeniable, with marked reductions in the number of movements or marked slowness of movement; subject rarely spontaneously moves or speaks. Hyperactivity is undeniable; subject moves almost constantly; in both cases, exam is prolonged as a consequence.)

a b c ☐ 3: severe (Hypoactivity is severe; patient does not move or speak without prodding or is catatonic. Hyperactivity is severe; patient is constantly moving, overreacts to stimuli, requires surveillance and/or restraint; getting through the exam is difficult or impossible.)

ITEM 10—SLEEP-WAKE CYCLE DISTURBANCE (DISORDER OR AROUSAL): Rate patient's ability to either sleep or stay awake at the appropriate times.

Utilize direct observation during the interview, as well as reports from nurses, family, patient, or charts describing sleep-wake cycle disturbance over the past several hours or since last examination. Use observations of the previous night for morning evaluations only.

☐ 0: none (at night, sleeps well; during the day, has no trouble staying awake)

☐ 1: mild (mild deviation from appropriate sleepfulness and wakefulness states; at night, difficulty falling asleep or transient night awakenings, needs medication to sleep well; during the day, reports

(continued)

Box 1.1 (Continued)

periods of drowsiness or, during the interview, is drowsy but can easily fully awaken him/herself)

☐ 2: moderate (moderate deviations from appropriate sleepfulness and wakefulness states; at night, repeated and prolonged night awakening; during the day, reports of frequent and prolonged napping or, during the interview, can only be roused to complete wakefulness by strong stimuli)

☐ 3: severe (severe deviations from appropriate sleepfulness and wakefulness states; at night, sleeplessness; during the day, patient spends most of the time sleeping or, during the interview, cannot be roused to full wakefulness by any stimuli)

Adapted from Breitbart W, Rosenfeld B, Roth A, Smith MJ, Cohen K, Passik S. The Memorial Delirium Assessment Scale. *J Pain & Sympt Manage*. Mar 1997;13(3):128–137.

Box 1.2 Short Michigan Alcoholism Screening Instrument—Geriatric Version (SMAST-G)

SMAST-G

1. When talking with others, do you ever underestimate how much you drink?

2. After a few drinks, have you sometimes not eaten or been able to skip a meal because you didn't feel hungry?

3. Does having a few drinks help decrease your shakiness or tremors?

4. Does alcohol sometimes make it hard for you to remember parts of the day or night?

5. Do you usually take a drink to relax or calm your nerves?

6. Do you drink to take your mind off your problems?

7. Have you ever increased your drinking after experiencing a loss in your life?

8. Has a doctor or nurse ever said they were worried or concerned about your drinking?

9. Have you ever made rules to manage your drinking?

10. When you feel lonely, does having a drink help?

(2 or more Yes responses are indicative of an alcohol problem)

Adapted from Blow FC GB, Barry KL, Mudd SA, Hill EM. Brief screening for alcohol problems in the elderly populations using the Short Michigan Alcoholism Screening Test-Geriatric Version (SMAST-G). *Alcohol Clin Exp Res*. 1998;22(Suppl: 131A).

CAGE Questions

Substance use is evaluated to assess substance abuse or dependence. The CAGE questions (Box 1.3) help guide the assessment of alcohol abuse. CAGE is an acronym for the four questions shown in the box.[14] A yes answer to at least two of these questions suggests alcohol abuse or dependence and should be considered clinically significant.

Box 1.3 CAGE Questions

1. Have you ever felt the need to **C**ut down?

   Yes   No

2. Do you get **A**nnoyed when other people are critical of your drinking?

   Yes   No

3. Do you feel **G**uilty about using?

   Yes   No

4. Have you ever needed an **E**ye-opener in the morning?

   Yes   No

Adapted from Ewing JA. Detecting alcoholism. The CAGE questionnaire. *JAMA*. Oct 12 1984;252(14):1905–1907.

Box 1.4 FICA Spiritual History Tool

F—Faith and Belief

Do you consider yourself spiritual or religious?" or "Do you have spiritual beliefs that help you cope with stress?" If the patient responds no, the health-care provider might ask, "What gives your life meaning?" Sometimes patients respond with answers such as family, career, or nature.

I—Importance

"What importance does your faith or belief have in our life? Have your beliefs influenced how you take care of yourself in this illness? What role do your beliefs play in regaining your health?"

C—Community

"Are you part of a spiritual or religious community? Is this of support to you and how? Is there a group of people you really love or who are important to you?" Communities such as churches, temples, and mosques, or a group of like-minded friends can serve as strong support systems for some patients.

A—Address in Care

"How would you like me, your health-care provider, to address these issues in your healthcare?"

Adapted from Puchalski C, Romer AL. Taking a spiritual history allows clinicians to understand patients more fully. *J Palliat Med.* Spring 2000;3(1):129–137.

Spirituality

FICA Spiritual History Tool

Spirituality is an important part of many people's lives and provides a sense of connectedness and comfort during times of illness and distress. Cancer often precipitates a spiritual crisis as a person searches for meaning in their life and illness. Spirituality is evaluated by questions surrounding four main themes to guide the clinician's history taking and provide a better sense of the patient's dependence on spirituality in coping with illness (Box 1.4). The questions are not scored but rather focus on strengths.[15]

References

1. *Screening tools for measuring distress* [CD-Rom]. Jenkintown, PA: National Comprehensive Cancer Network; May 2005.

2. Lyness JM, Noel TK, Cox C, King DA, Conwell Y, Caine ED. Screening for depression in elderly primary care patients. a comparison of the Center for Epidemiologic Studies-Depression Scale and the Geriatric Depression Scale. *Arch Intern Med.* Feb 24 1997;157(4):449–454.

3. Blazer DG. Depression in late life: review and commentary. *J Gerontol. Series A, Biological Sciences and Medical Sciences.* Mar 2003;58(3):249–265.

4. Morley JE. The top 10 hot topics in aging. *J.Gerontol. Series A, Biological Sciences and Medical Sciences.* Jan 2004;59(1):24–33.

5. Langa KM, Valenstein MA, Fendrick AM, Kabeto MU, Vijan S. Extent and cost of informal caregiving for older Americans with symptoms of depression. *Am J Psychiat.* May 2004;161(5):857–863.

6. Zigmond AS, Snaith RP. The hospital anxiety and depression scale. *Acta psychiatrica Scandinavica.* June 1983;67(6):361–370.

7. Folstein MF, Folstein SE, McHugh PR. "Mini-mental state." a practical method for grading the cognitive state of patients for the clinician. *J Psychiatr Res.* Nov 1975;12(3):189–198.

8. Katzman R, Brown T, Fuld P, Peck A, Schechter R, Schimmel H. Validation of a short Orientation-Memory-Concentration Test of cognitive impairment. *Am J Psychiat.* June 1983;140(6):734–739.

9. Juby A, Tench S, Baker V. The value of clock drawing in identifying executive cognitive dysfunction in people with a normal Mini-Mental State Examination score. *CMAJ: Canadian Medical Association Journal.* Oct 15 2002;167(8):859–864.

10. Watson YI, Arfken CL, Birge SJ. Clock completion: an objective screening test for dementia. *J Am Geriatr Soc.* Nov 1993;41(11):1235–1240.

11. Sunderland T, Hill JL, Mellow AM, et al. Clock drawing in Alzheimer's disease. A novel measure of dementia severity. *J Am Geriatr Soc.* Aug 1989;37(8):725–729.

12. Breitbart W, Rosenfeld B, Roth A, Smith MJ, Cohen K, Passik S. The Memorial Delirium Assessment Scale. *J Pain & Sympt Manage.* Mar 1997;13(3):128–137.

13. Blow FC GB, Barry KL, Mudd SA, Hill EM. Brief screening for alcohol problems in the elderly populations using the Short Michigan Alcoholism Screening Test-Geriatric Version (SMAST-G). *Alcohol Clin Exp Res.* 1998;22(Suppl: 131A).

14. Ewing JA. Detecting alcoholism. The CAGE questionnaire. JAMA. Oct 12 1984;252(14):1905–1907.

15. Puchalski C, Romer AL. Taking a spiritual history allows clinicians to understand patients more fully. *J Palliat Med.* Spring 2000;3(1):129–137.

16. Sheikh JI YJ. Geriatric Depression Scale (GDS): recent evidence and development of a shorter version. *J Clin Gerontol & Geriatr.* 1986;5(1/2):165–173.

Chapter 2

Functional Assessment for Older Adults with Cancer

Tanya M. Wildes

Introduction

Function refers to an individual's ability to perform particular tasks. It is influenced not only by the presence and severity of symptoms, but also by other internal and external factors, such as personal motivation and social/economic supports.[1] It influences, but is not synonymous with, health-related quality of life. In this chapter, we will discuss measures of functional status which are most commonly used in geriatric oncology, and discuss their utility and limitations in the care of older adults with cancer.

Performance Status

The need to describe a patient's function was addressed in the field of oncology with a construct known as performance status. The two most widely used instruments include the Eastern Cooperative Oncology Group (ECOG) performance status and the Karnofsky Performance Status[2] (Table 2.1). Performance status is commonly included in eligibility criteria for clinical trials, and is prognostic when used in routine clinical practice.

Activities of Daily Living and Instrumental Activities of Daily Living

The Index of Activities of Daily Living (ADLs) was developed by Katz et al. 50 years ago as a measure of function.[3] It was originally developed to be scored by an observer, but is now generally reported by the individual or caregiver. ADLs can be thought of as the activities required for an individual to remain independent within the home. The Instrumental Activities of Daily Living (IADLs) are the activities required for an individual to remain independent in the community. The Index of Instrumental Activities of Daily Living was similarly developed by Lawton and Brody, with a social worker obtaining the information from the "best available source" (subject, family, friends, or caregiver in an institution).[4] See Tables 2.2 and 2.3.

Table 2.1 Performance Status Measures

ECOG Performance Status		Karnofsky Performance Status	
0	Fully active, able to carry on all predisease performance without restriction	100	Normal; no complaints; no evidence of disease
		90	Able to carry on normal activity; minor signs of symptoms of disease
1	Restricted in physically strenuous activity but ambulatory and able to carry out work of a light or sedentary nature (e.g. light housework, office work)	80	Normal activity with effort; minor signs or symptoms of disease
		70	Cares for self but unable to carry on normal activity or to do active work
2	Ambulatory and capable of all self-care but unable to carry out any work activities. Up and about more than 50% of waking hours	60	Requires occasional assistance but is able to care for most of personal needs
		50	Requires considerable assistance and frequent medical care
3	Capable only of limited self-care, confined to bed or chair more than 50% of waking hours	40	Disabled; requires special care and assistance
		30	Severely disabled; hospitalization is indicated although death is not imminent.
4	Completely disabled. Cannot carry on any self-care. Totally confined to bed or chair	20	Very ill; hospitalization and active supportive care necessary
		10	Moribund
5	Dead	0	Dead

ECOG: Eastern Cooperative Oncology Group.

Adapted from Oken MM, Creech RH, Tormey DC, et al. Toxicity and response criteria of the Eastern Cooperative Oncology Group. *Am J Clin Oncol.* 1982 Dec;5(6):649–55.

Table 2.2 Katz Index of Activities of Daily Living

Assistance means supervision, direction or active personal assistance

Bathing—either sponge bath, tub bath or shower

- Receives no assistance (gets in and out of tub by self if tub is usual means of bathing)
- Receives assistance in bathing only one part of the body (such as back or leg)
- Receives assistance in bathing more than one part of the body (or not bathed)

Dressing—gets close from closet and drawers—including underclothes, outer garments and using fasteners (including braces if worn)

- Gets clothes and gets completely dressed without assistance
- Gets clothes and gets dressed without assistance except for assistance in tying shoes
- Receives assistance in getting clothes or in getting dressed, or stays partly or completely undressed

(continued)

Table 2.2 (Continued)

Toileting—goes to the "toilet room" for bowel and urine elimination; cleaning self after elimination, and arranging clothes

- Goes to the "toilet room, " cleans self and arranges clothes without assistance (may use object for support such as cane, walker or wheelchair and may manage night bedpan or commode, emptying same in the morning)
- Receives assistance in going to "toilet room" or in cleaning self or in arranging clothes after elimination or in use of night bedpan or commode
- Doesn't go to room termed "toilet" for elimination process

Transferring

- Moves in and out of bed as well as in and out of chair without assistance (may be using object for support such as cane or walker)
- Moves in and out of bed or chair with assistance
- Doesn't get out of bed

Continence

- Controls urination and bowel movement completely by self
- Has occasional "accidents"
- Supervision helps keep urine and bowel control; catheter is used, or is incontinent

Feeding

- Feeds self without assistance
- Feeds self except for getting assistance in cutting meat or buttering bread
- Receives assistance in feeding or is fed partly or completely by using tubes or intravenous fluids

Table 2.3 Lawton Index of Instrumental Activities of Daily Living

Ability to use telephone

- Operates telephone on own initiative—looks up and dials numbers, etc.
- Dials a few well-known numbers
- Answers telephone but does not dial
- Does not use telephone at all

Shopping

- Takes care of all shopping needs independently
- Shops independently for small purchases
- Needs to be accompanied on any shopping trip
- Completely unable to shop

Food preparation

- Plans, prepares and serves adequate meals independently
- Prepares adequate meals if supplied with ingredients
- Heats and serves prepared meals, or prepares meals but does not maintain an adequate diet
- Needs to have meals prepared and served

(continued)

...

Table 2.3 (Continued)

Housekeeping

- Maintains house alone, or with occasional assistance (e.g., "heavy work-domestic help")
- Performs light daily tasks such as dishwashing, bedmaking
- Performs light daily tasks but cannot maintain acceptable level of cleanliness
- Needs help with all home maintenance tasks
- Does not participate in any housekeeping tasks

Laundry

- Does personal laundry completely
- Launders small items—rinses socks, stockings, etc.
- All laundry must be done by others

Transportation

- Travels independently on public transportation or drives own car
- Arranges own travel via taxi, but does not otherwise use public transportation
- Travels on public transportation when assisted or accompanied by another
- Travel limited to taxi or automobile with assistance of another
- Does not travel at all

Responsibility for own medications

- Is responsible for taking medication in correct dosages at correct time
- Takes responsibility if medication is prepared in advance in separate dosages
- Is not capable of dispensing own medications

Ability to handle finances

- Manages financial matters independently (budgets, writes checks, pays rent, bills, goes to bank), collects and keeps track of income
- Manages day-to-day purchases, but needs help with banking, major purchases, etc.
- Incapable of handling money

Physical Performance Measures

Objective, performance-based measures of physical performance can provide an additional measure of function. Physical performance tests correlate only moderately with self-report of function,[5] suggesting that, in some cases, physical performance measures may yield additional information. There are a number of validated physical performance measures; some predominantly assess lower extremity function, whereas others assess both upper and lower extremity function. Two physical performance tests commonly used in the geriatric oncology literature is the Timed Up and Go Test[6] and the Short Physical Performance Battery[7]. In the Timed Up and Go Test, subjects are timed as they rise from being seated in an armchair, walk 3 meters, turn and return to a seated position in the chair. The Short Physical Performance Battery assesses standing balance with a progressive Romberg, walking speed during a 2.4-meter walk, and the ability to rise from a chair 5 times. In community-dwelling populations, poorer performance on the SPPB predicts new disability at 4 years of follow-up.

Other Measures Are Not Surrogates for functional assessment

Clinicians unfamiliar with assessing older adults may mistakenly believe that information, such as age and comorbidities, gleaned in a routine history and physical exam may suffice for estimating function. However, this is not the case. In cohorts of older adults with cancer, age and ADL disability are *independent*, and age and IADL disability are only weakly correlated. Similarly, comorbidities and function are independent.[8] Thus, clinicians must explicitly ask about daily activities and dependence in order to have an accurate understanding of the patient's function.

Utility of Functional Assessment in Older Adults with Cancer

A growing body of literature is demonstrating that performance status alone is an inadequate measure of function in older adults with cancer, and that measures of ADL/IADL function are both predictive and prognostic. Performance status alone underestimates the level of disability in older adults with cancer. In a cross-sectional study of older adults with newly diagnosed cancer, among patients with a "good" performance status (ECOG 0–1), almost 10 percent were dependent in at least one ADL, and nearly 40 percent were dependent in one or more IADLs.[9]

Two recent studies demonstrated the predictive utility of functional status assessment. In the Cancer and Aging Research Group's multi-institutional prospective cohort study of 500 older adults with cancer receiving chemotherapy, IADL dependence (specifically, requiring assistance with taking medication) was independently associated with greater odds of severe toxicity of chemotherapy.[10] Notably, the Karnofsky Performance Status did not predict chemotherapy toxicity in this study. In the Chemotherapy Risk Assessment in High Age Patients (CRASH) study, Extermann et al. showed that dependence in IADLs was associated with greater risk of severe hematologic toxicity in older adults receiving chemotherapy, and that poorer performance status was associated with non-hematologic toxicity.[11] Dependence in IADLs is also predictive of surgical complications among older adults undergoing cancer surgery.[12]

Functional status is predictive of survival as well. A number of studies have demonstrated associations between poorer function and poorer survival.[13] In a prospective cohort study of older adults with cancer, slower time on the Timed Up and Go Test was associated with a two-and-a-half times greater odds of death in the first 6 months.[14] Such prognostic information may aid clinicians and patients tremendously, allowing patients with incurable malignancies to make more-informed decisions and to meet their goals of care by adding individualized, function-based prognostic information to cancer-related prognostic information.

Importance of Maintaining Functional Status

In addition to the utility of assessing functional status for predicting toxicity of chemotherapy and survival, functional independence is in and of itself important to patients. In a study of older adults with life-limiting illness, 70 percent of cancer patients reported that they would forgo a treatment that would result in severe functional impairment.[15] Thus, it is of utmost importance for a clinician to understand a patient's current level of function and their treatment preferences, and estimate the risk of therapy in order to inform shared decision making about cancer therapy.

Conclusions

Functional assessments of older adults with cancer are an essential part of their care. The information gained may guide discussions to help the older adult meet their goals of care, by providing information about risk of chemotherapy toxicity, surgical complications, and prognosis.

References

1. Wilson IB, Cleary PD. Linking clinical variables with health-related quality of life. A conceptual model of patient outcomes. *JAMA* 1995 Jan 4;273(1):59–65.

2. Oken MM, Creech RH, Tormey DC, et al. Toxicity and response criteria of the Eastern Cooperative Oncology Group. *Am J Clin Oncol*. 1982 Dec;5(6):649–655.

3. Katz S, Ford, AB, Moskowitz R, Jackson B, Jaffe M. Studies of illness in the aged: the index of ADL. *JAMA*. 1963;185:914–919.

4. Lawton M, Brody E. Assessment of older people: self-maintaining and instrumental activities of daily living. *Gerontologist*. 1969;9(3):179–986.

5. Sherman SE, Reuben D. Measures of functional status in community-dwelling elders. *J Gen Intern Med*. 1998 Dec;13(12):817–823.

6. Podsiadlo D, Richardson S. The timed "Up & Go": a test of basic functional mobility for frail elderly persons. *J Am Geriatr Soc*. 1991 Feb;39(2):142–148.

7. Guralnik JM, Ferrucci L, Simonsick EM, Salive ME, Wallace RB. Lower-extremity function in persons over the age of 70 years as a predictor of subsequent disability. *NEJM*. 1995 Mar 2;332(9):556–561.

8. Extermann M, Overcash J, Lyman GH, Parr J, Balducci L. Comorbidity and functional status are independent in older cancer patients. *J Clin. Oncol*. 1998 Apr;16(4):1582–1587.

9. Repetto L, Fratino L, Audisio RA, et al. Comprehensive geriatric assessment adds information to Eastern Cooperative Oncology Group performance status in elderly cancer patients: an Italian Group for Geriatric Oncology Study. *J. Clin. Oncol*. 2002 Jan 15;20(2):494–502.

10. Hurria A, Togawa K, Mohile SG, et al. Predicting chemotherapy toxicity in older adults with cancer: a prospective multicenter study. *J Clin Oncol*. 2011 Aug 30;29(25):3457–3465.

11. Extermann M, Boler I, Reich RR, et al. Predicting the risk of chemotherapy toxicity in older patients: The Chemotherapy Risk Assessment Scale for High-Age Patients (CRASH) score. *Cancer*. 2012 Jul 1;118(13):3377–3386.

12. Audisio RA, Ramesh H, Sestini A, et al. Shall we operate? Preoperative assessmentin elderly cancer patients (PACE) can help A SIOG surgical task force prospective study. *Crit Rev Oncol/Hematol*. 2008;65:156–163.

13. Puts M, Hardt J, Monette J, Girre V. Use of geriatric assessment for older adults in the oncology setting: a systematic review. *J Natl Cancer Inst*. 2012;1 04(15):1133–1163.

14. Soubeyran P, Fonck M, Blanc-Bisson C, et al. Predictors of early death risk in older patients treated with first-line chemotherapy for cancer. *J Clin Oncol*. 2012 May 20;30(15):1829–34.

15. Fried TR, Bradley EH, Towle VR, Allore H. Understanding the treatment preferences of seriously ill patients. *NEJM*. 2002 Apr 4;346(14):1061–1066.

Chapter 3

Psychosocial Interventions for Older Cancer Patients

Lea Baider, Talia Weiss Wiesel, and Jimmie C. Holland

Introduction

Elderly patients with cancer face unique physical and psychiatric challenges in coping with their illness. Common issues facing this population include depression and anxiety, demoralization and existential concerns, loneliness and isolation, and other quality-of-life problems.

There are few interventions specifically tailored to older adults with cancer.[1] However, several interventions that have proven effective in community-dwelling older adults and palliative-care patients may be adapted/modified for use in the geriatric oncology setting. This chapter describes two interventions developed specifically to address the issues older patients with cancer face and several interventions used with community-dwelling older adults and palliative-care patients.

Geriatric Oncology Specific Interventions

1. The CARE Intervention—Cancer and Aging: Reflections of Elders

This is a 6-session intervention, primarily cognitive based. CARE is grounded in an integration of Susan Folkman's cognitive coping paradigm, which utilizes reappraisal, and Erik Erikson's eighth and final psychosocial developmental life stage, in which the task is to achieve ego integrity (equanimity). This intervention is geared toward reducing depression, isolation, and despair related to the "double whammy" of aging and illness. The goal of CARE is to foster relatedness, acceptance of illness, and a sense of meaningful integration.[2,3]

CARE is currently nearing completion of a random controlled trial (RCT) comparing the intervention delivered over the phone (5 sessions over 7 weeks) with standard care at Memorial Sloan Kettering Cancer Center. Preliminary results suggest the CARE Intervention is feasible and effective; data shows a reduction in depression, anxiety demoralization, and loneliness. Patients also had an increase in spiritual well-being. At the last follow-up assessment, patients testimonials included: "I can laugh more than ever," "[I] have a better outlook on cancer, a way to reflect on disease and rest of life," and "Questions made [me] look back upon life and appreciate support and love [I] had." The intervention will be tested further in a face-to-face and online group model.

Group Session Topics Include:
- Coping with Cancer and Aging: Dealing with the combined problems of illness and aging utilizing life review.
- Facing the Unknowns of Cancer and Aging: Coping with concerns, worries, and fears of the future.
- Loneliness and The Stigma of Cancer and Aging: Loneliness and reduced social circles in later years.
- Making Peace with One's Life: Who Am I? Coming to terms with "Who I am now."
- Wisdom and the Keepers of Meaning: Contributing to the greater good, passing on one's worth and wisdom.

2. Coping and Communication Support for Older Cancer Patients (CCS)

Coping and Communication Support is a supportive intervention for older advanced stage patients and their family caregivers.[4] The intervention is delivered by nurses with mental health training and is delivered by telephone, e-mail, or clinic visit, according to patient preference. Patients and caregivers have a 24/7 direct telephone/e-mail access to their nurse. Patients remain in the intervention until death, and their caregivers remain in for one or more years to ensure an easy bereavement.

Frame
- Initial follow-up contact is made within 2 weeks of the initial meeting.
- A patient with high distress (DT ≥ 4) is contacted minimally on a monthly basis unless the participant has expressed preference for less frequent contact.

CCS Functions
- Facilitation of patient goals.
- Assistance with resolution of problems.
- Assistance with navigating the healthcare system.
- Support of the patient, as requested.
- Communicating with physicians.

CCS Components
- Patients develops the agenda.
- Respects the participants' emotional boundaries.
- Identifies the participants' preference for future contact.
- Considers the participants' preference for problem identification.

3. Improving Mood Promoting Access to Collaborative Treatment (IMPACT) Program

The IMPACT program is a stepped care-management program for depression in primary-care patients who had an ICD-9 cancer diagnosis.[5] Fann conducted an RCT in which intervention patients had access for up to

12 months to a depression-care manager who was supervised by a psychiatrist and a primary-care provider and who offered education; care management; support of antidepressant management; and brief, structured psychosocial interventions including behavioral activation and problem-solving treatment. At 6 and 12 months, intervention patients had a significant reduction in depressive symptoms and a significant improvement in quality of life. Intervention patients also experienced greater remission rates, more depression-free days, and less functional impairment.

Providers
- Depression care manager (DCM).
  - Nurse.
  - Clinical psychologist.

Intervention
- Psychosocial history.
- Psycho-education.
- Behavioral activation (which emphasizes pleasant event scheduling and overcoming avoidance behaviors).
- Aid patients in identifying treatment preferences.
- Treatment options:
  - Antidepressant medicines prescribed by the patients' primary-care clinicians.
  - Structured 6–8-session psychotherapy program: Problem-Solving Treatment (PST).
- The DCM met weekly with a supervising psychiatrist and an expert primary-care physician (PCP) to monitor clinical progress and adjust treatment plans accordingly.
- In-person or telephone follow-up visits occurred ~every 2 weeks during acute-phase treatment, with subsequent monthly contact during continuation and maintenance phases.
- The intervention did not include routine assessment or treatment of cancer-related issues, although patients could choose to address cancer-related problems in PST sessions.

Geriatric

1. Supportive Psychotherapy
Supportive psychotherapy is an intervention that helps patients deal with distress, reinforce preexisting strengths, and promote adaptive coping with illness.[6] It explores the patient's self, body image, and role changes within a relationship of mutual respect and trust.

Therapeutic Approach
- Clarify and discuss highly charged information, which arouses overwhelming emotions that interfere with function, and help to manage these emotions constructively.
- Problem solving.

- Being comfortable with a range of therapeutic activity including crisis intervention and a quiet, supportive presence for patients too weak to interact, an exploration of deep dynamic patterns operating in the patient's psyche and family counseling.
- Standing ready to guide the patient and family to available resources.
- Working with the medical caregivers and understanding the system in which they operate to allow the reciprocal flow of useful information. This means knowing how to discuss the coping abilities and the vulnerabilities of the patient, in ways that humanize without violating confidentiality.
- Understanding the medical information you are given, and asking if you need more help.
- Understanding your own emotional responses, especially in your early years as you learn to manage yourself for the long haul, in these demanding situations.

Themes in Advanced Cancer
- Family legacies.
  - The meaning of cancer.
  - The meaning of illness.
- Guilt.
- Fear of death.
- Spirituality and religion in supportive therapy.
- Transition to palliative care.
- End of life.

2. Mindfulness-Based Stress Reduction and Relaxation Interventions

Mindfulness-Based Stress Reduction (MBSR) is an intervention developed by Jon Kabbat-Zinn and has been adapted for people with cancer (*Mindfulness-Based Cancer Recovery*). Mindfulness is "paying attention in a particular way: on purpose, in the present moment and nonjudgmentally."[7] Relaxation consists of learning different ways to reduce the body's stress response in order to induce the "relaxation response."

Mindfulness Treatment
- Body scan.
- Mindfulness meditation.
- Informal mindfulness.
- Breathing.

Relaxation Treatment
- Guided imagery.
- Visualization.
- Progressive muscular relaxation.
- Deep breathing.
- Cue controlled relaxation.

Goals of Relaxation
- Support and promote:
  - Well-being and coping.

- Control and mastery
- Coping skills for treatment-related side effects and procedure-related distress.
- Prevent distress.

3. Cognitive Behavioral Therapy

The goal of Cognitive Behavioral Therapy (CBT) is to understand how a patient's unhelpful thinking styles (distorted thinking) adversely affect their ability to cope with stressful life events, and to aid the patient in their ability to identify *cognitive distortions* in their *automatic thoughts*, to *critically evaluate* these distortions, challenge them and create *adaptive responses*.[8]

CBT enables patients to
- Change their emotional and behavioral responses to the events of their illness through a process of re-learning.
- Replace dysfunctional thoughts with adaptive ones.
- See a direct connection between thoughts, feelings, and behavior.
- Create a new, more functional way of thinking.

Common Cognitive Distortions and Misinterpretations of Reality
1. **All-or-Nothing Thinking:** seeing things in black and white categories.
2. **Overgeneralization:** seeing a single negative event as a never-ending pattern.
3. **Mental Filters:** picking a single negative detail and dwelling on it exclusively, so that your vision of all reality becomes darkened.
4. **Disqualifying the Positive:** rejecting positive experiences by insisting "they don't count" for some reason or other.
5. **Jumping to Conclusions:** making a negative interpretation even though there are no facts that support the conclusion.
   a. **Mind Reading:** arbitrarily concluding someone is reacting negatively to you.
   b. **Fortune Telling:** anticipating things will turn out badly.
6. **Magnification or Minimizing:** exaggerating the importance of things (e.g., your own goof up) or inappropriately shrinking things (e.g., your own desirable qualities).
7. **Emotional Reasoning:** assuming your negative emotions necessarily reflect the way things really are.
8. **"Should" Statements**: "I should be able to feel better by now." Statements that place additional burden on the patient not necessarily reflecting the reality.
9. **Labeling or Mislabeling:** an extreme form of overgeneralization (e.g., "I'm a loser").
10. **Personalization:** seeing yourself as the cause of a negative external event for which you're not primarily responsible.

Typical Structure of a CBT Session
- Agenda setting.
- Working systematically through a problem.

- Summarizing.
- Eliciting feedback.

3. Interpersonal Psychotherapy (IPT)

IPT is a time-limited (16 sessions) therapy with four possible foci, based on a medical model of depression. IPT places an emphasis on the link between patients' depressed mood and *current* interpersonal relations. The goals are to reduce depressive symptoms and improve interpersonal functioning.[9]

Three Phases of IPT
1. Initial (sessions 1–3).
2. Intermediate (sessions 4–13).
3. Termination (sessions 14–16).

Four Foci
- Interpersonal disputes—conflicts with a significant other.
- Role transition—any change in life status.
- Grief—"complicated bereavement" following death of loved one.
- Interpersonal deficits—lack of social skills.

Therapeutic Techniques
- Reassurance.
- Identification and exploration of emotions.
- Encouragement of affect.
- Amelioration of communication with others (communication analysis).
- Role-playing.
- Encouragement of behavior change.
- Use of therapeutic relationship.

Palliative

1. Meaning-Centered Psychotherapy

This existential-based intervention is based on the works of Viktor Frankl and Irvin Yalom, geared toward advanced cancer patients.[10] The goal is to diminish despair, demoralization, hopelessness, and a desire for hastened death by sustaining or enhancing a sense of meaning, even in the face of death. The intervention has two forms: individual (7 one-hour sessions) and group (8 one-and-a-half-hour sessions).

Session Structure
- Process last session.
- Introduction to session topic.
- Experiential exercise.
- Review of homework assignment for following session.

Session Topics
1. Concepts and sources of meaning.
   a. Introductions.
   b. Introduction of concept and sources of meaning.

2. Cancer and meaning.
   a. Identity before and after cancer diagnosis.
3. Historical sources of meaning.
   a. Life as a legacy that has been given (past).
   b. Life as a legacy that one lives (present).
   c. Life as a legacy that one gives (future).
4. Attitudinal sources of meaning: encountering life's limitations.
   a. Confronting the limitations imposed by cancer, prognosis, and death.
   b. Introduction to legacy project.
5. Creative sources of meaning: engaging in life fully.
   a. Creativity, courage, responsibility.
6. Experiential Sources of Meaning.
   a. Love, nature, art, and humor.
7. Transitions
   a. Review of sources of meaning, as resources, reflections on lessons learned in treatment.

2. Dignity Therapy

Dignity therapy is a patient affirming psychotherapeutic intervention addressing existential and psychosocial distress in advanced stage patients.[11] The goal is to improve quality of life through reflection and introspection of life events, thoughts, feelings, values, and life accomplishments.

Benefits
- Spiritual and psychological well-being.
- Reducing suffering.
- Increase meaning and purpose.

Dignity Therapy Questions
- Tell me a little about your life history, particularly the parts that you either remember the most or those you think are the most important?
- When did you feel most alive?
- Are there particular things that you would want your family to know about you, and are there particular things you would want them to remember?
- What are the most important roles you have played in your life (family, vocational, community service roles, etc.)? Why were they so important to you, and what do you think you accomplished within those roles?
- What are your most important accomplishments, and what do you feel most proud of? Alternately, what do you take pride in?
- Are there particular things that you feel need to be said to your loved ones or things you would want to take the time to say once again?
- What are your hopes and dreams for your loved ones?
- What have you learned about life that you would want to pass along to others? What advice or words of guidance would you wish to pass along to your (son, daughter, spouse, parents, and other(s))?

Dignity Themes

A. Illness-related concerns.
　1. Level of independence.
　　a. Cognitive acuity.
　　b. Functional capacity.
　2. Symptom distress.
　　a. Physical distress.
　　b. Psychological distress.
　　　i. Medical uncertainty.
　　　ii. Death anxiety.
B. Dignity-conserving repertoire.
　1. Dignity-conserving perspectives.
　　a. Continuity of self.
　　b. Role preservation.
　　c. Generativity/legacy (e.g., "What will I leave behind for my family/ for my community?").
　　d. Maintenance of pride.
　　e. Hopefulness.
　　f. Autonomy/control.
　　g. Acceptance.
　　h. Resilience/fighting spirit.
　2. Dignity-conserving practices.
　　a. Living "in the moment."
　　b. Maintaining normalcy.
　　c. Seeking spiritual comfort.
C. Social-dignity inventory.
　1. Privacy boundaries.
　2. Social support.
　3. Care tenor.
　4. Burden to others.
　5. Aftermath concerns.

3. Family Therapy at the End of Life

Family-focused grief therapy (FFGT) is focused and time-limited, consisting of six to ten 90-minute sessions arranged across 9–18 months.[12] FFGT is a manualized intervention aimed to optimize cohesion, communication (of thoughts and feelings), and the handling of conflict while promoting the sharing of grief and mutual support.

Phases of FFGT

1. Assessment phase (1–2 weekly sessions).
2. Intervention (3–6 monthly sessions).
3. Termination (1–2 sessions spaced 2–3 months apart as booster sessions).

Phase 1: Assessment
- Welcome and orientation.
- Data gathering:
  - Story of illness.
  - Communication.
  - Cohesiveness.
  - Conflict.
  - Roles, rules, and expectations.
  - Values and beliefs.
- Construct family genome, seek to understand coping patterns with previous losses and relational styles across generations.
- Identify family strengths.
- Summarize family concerns in the context of their functioning.
- Clarify options and agree on future management plan.

Phase 2: Focused Treatment
- Welcome and orientation.
- Review how family is coping with illness and grief over losses or bereavement.
- Acknowledge losses and related grief, including any emergent strength in mutual support.
- Remind the family of their prioritized concerns, including relevant aspects of communication, cohesiveness, and conflict resolution, or otherwise agreed targets of the work.
- Unspoken concerns/palliative care themes.
- Summarize what progress is evident, affirming strengths alongside any continuing targets for future effort.
- Arrange next session, locating it within the overall plan of time-limited therapy.

Key Theoretical Models underpinning FFGT
- Attachment theory.
- Cognitive-processing theory.
- Group adaptation.

Key Therapeutic Processes
- Facilitating talk about death and dying.
- Talk about prognosis.
- Talk about "Talk" (i.e., discussing the process of talking together about illness).
- Talk about future needs.

Non-Evidence-Based Geriatric Oncology Interventions

1. Reminiscence/Life Review

The functions of reminiscence/life review therapy are to:[13] come to terms with age, accept difficult aspects of their past, resolve past conflicts, make peace with the discrepancy between ideal and reality, examine of the past, recall the coping strategies used to get through difficult times, and empower patients to believe they can overcome the challenges of aging and illness. Sessions involve looking at old photographs to foster memories, audio-taping one's autobiography, attending reunions, constructing a genealogy, and music listening.

2. Forgiveness

Forgiveness Intervention for Older Cancer Patients

Forgiveness therapy has been shown to be effective in improving psychological well-being in older palliative care patients, specifically in the domains of hope, quality of life, and anger.[14] The content of the intervention addresses the patient's personal stories of perceived unjust and deep hurt. Forgiveness is offered as a healthy alternative to the negative emotions being experienced by the patient.

Components of the Intervention Sessions

- *Uncovering phase:* The patient reveals insights about how injustices and subsequent injuries have compromised their life.
- *Decision Phase:* The patient is given a choice to let go of the pain that he or she had carried for years. A decision to forgive is a cognitive process. Forgiveness is not complete in this stage.
- *Work phase:* The one forgiving may begin to experience some self-compassion.
- *Deepening phase:* Insights often stimulate other thoughts, such as "Have I needed others' forgiveness in the past?"

Conclusions

Elderly patients with cancer face unique physical and psychiatric challenges in coping with their illness, reviewed in Chapter 3 Impact of Aging on Cancer. Interventions specifically tailored to older adults with cancer were reviewed as well as several interventions, which have proven effective in community dwelling older adults and palliative-care patients, which may be adapted/modified for use in the geriatric oncology setting.

References

1. Baider L, Balducci L. Psychosocial interventions for elderly cancer patients: how old would you be if you did notknow how old you are?, In: Watson M, Kissane D, eds. *Handbook of Psychotherapy in Cancer Care*. Hoboken, NJ: Wiley-Blackwell; 2011: pp. 235–246.

2. Holland J, Poppito S, Nelson C, et al. Reappraisal in the eighth life cycle stage: a theoretical psychoeducational intervention in elderly patients with cancer. *Palliat and Support Care*. 2009;7:271–279.

3. Roth A, Napolitano S, Kenowitz J, et al. The cáncer and aging: reflection for elders (CARE) intervention. Presented at the APOS 9th Annual Conference, Miami, FL, February 2012.

4. Radziewicz RM, Rose JH, Bowman KF, et al. Establishing treatment fidelity in a coping and communication support telephone intervention for aging patients with advanced cancer and their family caregivers. *Cancer Nurs.* 2009;32:193–202.

5. Fann JR, Fan MY, Unützer J: Improving primary care for older adults with cancer and depression. *J Gen Intern Med.* 2009;24:417–24.

6. Lederberg MS, Holland JC: Supportive psychotherapy in cancer care: an essential ingredient of all therapy. In: Watson M, Kissane D., eds, *Handbook of Psychotherapy in Cancer Care.* Oxford, UK: Wiley-Blackwell: 2011.

7. Payne DK. Mindfulness intervention for cancer patients. In Watson M, Kissane D, eds., *Handbook of Psychotherapy in Cancer Care.* Oxford, UK: Wiley-Blackwell; 2011.

8. Laidlaw K, Thompson LW, Siskin LD: *Cognitive Behavior Therapy with Older People.* New York, NY: Wiley; 2003.

9. Hinrichsen GA, Clougherty KF: Interpersonal psychotherapy for depressed older adults. Washington, DC: American Psychological Association; 2006.

10. Breitbart W, Applebaum A: *Meaning-Centered Group Psychotherapy, in Watson M, Kissane D (eds): Handbook of Psychotherapy in Cancer Care.* Oxford, UK: Wiley-Blackwell; 2011.

11. Chochinov HM, McKeen. NA: Dignity therapy. In: Watson M, Kissane D, eds., *Handbook of Psychotherapy in Cancer Care.* Oxford, UK: Wiley-Blackwell: 2011.

12. Kissane DW, Zaider TI: Focused family therapy in palliative care and bereavment. In: Watson M, Kissane D, eds., *Handbook of Psychotherapy in Cancer Care.* Oxford, UK: Wiley-Blackwell; 2011.

13. Cappeliez P, Robitaille A. Coping mediates the relationships between reminiscence and psychological well-being among older adults. *Aging and Mental Health.* 2010;14:807–818.

14. Hansen MJ, Enright RD, Baskin TW, et al. A palliative care intervention in forgiveness therapy for elderly terminally ill cancer patients. *J Palliat Care.* 2009;25:51–60.

Psychiatric Emergencies and Disorders

Chapter 4

Psychiatric Emergencies

Andrew J. Roth

How does an oncology team handle a psychiatric emergency when a psychiatric consultant is not available? *First priority: safety of the patient and anyone else in danger. Managing emergencies in older cancer patients requires knowledge of their unique medical and psychiatric circumstances that will lead to accurate diagnoses and appropriate interventions.* See Box 4.1 and Table 4.1.

Interventions

Several steps may be taken to calm the patient. If needed, medication may be used to tranquilize the patient. An algorithm for medication is provided in Figure 4.1, and guidance on application of the algorithm may be found in Table 4.2. Also see Box 4.2.

Management of a Suicidal Emergency

Assessment of Risk

Suicidal thoughts are frightening for the patient, family, and the medical staff, although they are common and may be an attempt at feeling more psychological control over an uncertain future. Figuring out if someone is in acute danger of self-destructive behavior is not always easy. An older patient may be thinking, "I've lived a long life; if *it* gets bad enough, then I will kill myself." Most patients do not want to die and probably will not harm themselves but, rather, wish to share their frustration and fears about their situation. Older men are among the highest risk of patients who will

---

Box 4.1 Who Are the Patients Who Require Urgent Management?

- Patients who are violent, confused, hallucinating or suicidal.
- Patients who have questionable decisional capacity to refuse appropriate urgent treatment.
- Patients who are *restless, pacing, threatening, demanding, and/or pulling out tubes.*

Table 4.1 Management Principles for Psychiatric Emergencies in Older Patients

Safety First: How can the patient be safe, watched, and assessed? The answer depends on the setting.	• In the *hospital*, call a security officer. Does the patient need an order for one-to-one constant observation for safety by nursing personnel or security? Tell the patient you will call a family member to come in to be a support for the patient.
	• In the *clinic*, is there sufficient staff or assistance to monitor and control the patient's behavior? If not, consider transfer to an emergency room for medical clearance and call 911.
	• If at *home*, can family bring the patient to clinic or Emergency Room? If not, call 911 or police to take the patient to the nearest emergency room.
Obtain information from chart, staff, and family as quickly as possible. It is difficult, and sometimes dangerous, to assume what the baseline mental status is in an older patient.	• It is most ideal to gather emergency contacts for each patient (family, friends, and nursing home staff) before the occurrence of any emergency. Obtain advanced directives and health care proxy (HCP) designation for every patient early on in treatment and at the beginning of any hospitalization.
	• What is the behavior creating the emergency?
	• Try to ascertain the patient's baseline mental status from family, friends, or staff familiar with the patient.
	• Has the patient been agitated, confused, suicidal, or violent before?
	• Assess the mental status of the patient: is s/he disoriented, delusional, hallucinating, or psychotic?
	• What is the timeframe for the change in behavior or cognition?
	• What is the medical status of the patient?
	• Is there any history of alcohol or substance use or abuse? Could this be related to withdrawal? Just because the patient is older doesn't mean this can be disregarded.
	• What is your working differential diagnosis?
	• Have there been any recent medical or surgical procedures or changes in baseline medications? Consider polypharmacy interactions.
Take charge.	• The key to handling a psychiatric emergency in an elderly cancer patient is to *identify one person who is in charge*, preferably the oncologist. Emotions are high, and a single individual should direct the management of the emergency. Your calm stance is critical to safety for the patient, family, staff, and other bystanders who are frightened by disruptive behavior. Be respectful (use formal salutations "Mr. or Ms. or Dr." rather than first names unless you are familiar with the patient and speak to them in this informal nature.

(continued)

Table 4.1 (Continued)

	• Enlist someone the patient trusts, either a familiar staff member or family, to reassure the patient.
	• Give clear and concise instructions to all involved.
	• Get a language interpreter if appropriate.
	• Ask for psychiatric assistance if needed.
Work-up	• Assume a medical cause of agitation or confusion until proven otherwise, but keep psychogenic causes in mind if the medical options are ruled out.
	• Agitation or confusion may signal a medical emergency.
Being prepared	• Develop a "psychiatric code" procedure for psychiatric emergencies and practice it periodically with the multidisciplinary team, including security. Review safety issues that are particular to older patients.
	• Useful institutional phone numbers should be kept on hand and easily available:
	• Hospital Security, 911, or police
	• Psychiatrist on call
	• Emergency Room
	• Chaplaincy
	• Social Work
	• Psychiatric hospital admission contact
	• Language interpreters/translators
Physical restraint: Restraint entails holding a patient to lead them to a safe environment or while dispensing emergent medications, or when using 2- or 4-point limb restraints to restrict movement for extended periods of time to keep the patient and others safe.	• Enough well-trained staff is necessary to secure each limb. Four security guards or strong staff members may be needed to escort the patient.
	• Older patients are frail, have coagulation impairments, and possibly fragile bones because of age and cancer sequelae—If needed for safety, they must be physically restrained with care.
	• Physical restraints are used as briefly as possible, usually with either 2-point (arms) or 4-point (arms and legs) restraint devices.
	• Four-point restraints require checks every 15 minutes; a physician's order must be renewed every 4 hours. The patient remains under one-to-one constant observation status while 4-point restraints are in use. Ensure adequate hydration status.
	• Vital signs should be checked frequently and restraint sites rotated.
	• Frequent reorientation and explanation of what is happening should be communicated to the patient.
	• Each institution may have distinct legal policies.

(continued)

Table 4.1 (Continued)

Medication to tranquilize	See Figure 4.1 for algorithm for medicating agitated patients. • Inject a tranquilizer as needed (intravenous or intramuscular) when the patient is restrained if the cause of agitation is clear and not from an undiagnosed medical problem, or to facilitate a medical work-up. Intravenous administration is preferred given coagulopathies and potential decreased muscle mass in the elderly. • Psychotropic medications should not be used as chemical restraints to "keep patients quiet." • A useful rule of thumb when medicating older patients with cancer is: **Start low (dose), go slowly . . . but go (as needed).** • **Traditional antipsychotics (preferred given cardiovascular warnings about atypical antipsychotics and parenteral options)**—haloperidol (Haldol®), chlorpromazine (Thorazine®). • **Atypical antipsychotics**—olanzapine (Zyprexa®), risperidone (Risperdal®), quetiapine (Seroquel®), ziprasidone (Geodon®). • **Benzodiazepines**—lorazepam (Ativan®), diazepam (Valium®) (IV and PO), clonazepam (Klonopin), alprazolam (Xanax®) (PO). • **Benzodiazepines** can cause intoxication and delirium in elderly, cognitively compromised patients in particular. They but may be useful for acute sedation, or for agitated delirious patients, but should be given with neuroleptics in this population. After the patient is calm, the medical evaluation needs to be expedited. • Continue to observe the patient closely for safety and for the need of more medication. • Tranquilizers are sometimes continued until the cause has been reversed; observe vital signs regularly, as well as signs of parkinsonism, electrocardiogram QTc prolongation, mental status and cognitive changes, and neuroleptic malignant syndrome (NMS). If benzodiazepines are used, monitor respiratory status.

complete suicides, and have often told some physician their thoughts sometime before the suicide attempt. (See Chapter 6, Depressive Spectrum Disorders.)

Assessment of patients' intent and plans to hurt themselves is vital, understanding that sometimes the most vulnerable person may be the one who will not tell you what they are planning.

Box 4.2 Calming the Agitated Patient

- Start by talking to the patient to calm excited behavior.
- Isolate the patient away from other patients and visitors in the hospital or clinic.
- If in the hospital, escort the patient to a quiet room, with security, if needed, away from other patients.
- Determine whether family or friends are helping to calm the patient or agitating further. Enlist their help if they understand the situation. Call a trusted family member in to the hospital or clinic if they are not already present.
- Identify the staff member the patient trusts (e.g., male, female, older, younger, and trusted before); ask staff members who are the target of the patient's paranoia not to participate temporarily.
- Offer the "non-choice choice": Tell the patient they may choose what to do. "You can take the haloperidol (Haldol®) liquid, a calming medication, by mouth or we can give you an injection of Haldol®, either in a muscle or by the IV. Which would you rather have?"
- Or you may say, "We can all walk to your room and you can lie down, or the security guards can escort you to your room." Each time, you offer a less or more intrusive and coercive choice. The more rational the patient's thinking, the more likely s/he will choose the less intrusive option.
- Calm, concise explanations help the patient to cooperate. Allow the patient to express his concerns and frustrations in order to reduce the fears and lack of cooperation.

Examples of Expressions of Suicide, Which Are Not Usually Accompanied by High Risk

- "I've dealt with this illness for so many years, and I'm old; I will die of something sometime. I don't think I can go through another procedure and would rather die."
- "This may be a new diagnosis, but it is Cancer. If the pain ever gets bad enough, I will kill myself."

Examples of Expressions with Greater Suicidal Risk

- "This pain is unbearable. There's no way I can go on living like this."
- The patient has a gun at home.
- "Everyone would be better off without me."
- The patient is stockpiling pills.

The seriousness of the patient's intentions should be explored. Suicide occurs in patients with depression, severe anxiety, panic, intoxication, or delirium. *It is important to ask if the patient has made a definite plan.* See Tables 4.3 and 4.4.

	Hypoactive Delirium	OR SWITCH TO →	Hyperactive Delirium	OR SWITCH TO ←→	Hyperactive Delirium
MEDICATION:	Haloperidol		Chlorpromazine		Olanzapine
APPROXIMATE DAILY DOSE:	0.5–10 mg Q2–12 hr		25–50 mg IV Q4h–12 hr if increased sedation desired OR if haloperidol or olanzapine regimen is not tolerated		2.5–5 mg if EPS is a concern or if increased sedation desired OR if haloperidol or chlorpromazine regimen is not tolerated
ROUTE:	IV, IM, PO		IV, IM, PO		PO, IM or Zydis wafer
NEED TO WATCH FOR:	Extrapyramidal symptoms (EPS), EKG		EKG abnormalities, BP		Anticholinergic side effects
	If EPS is present, add benztropine 0.5–1 mg		Liver function tests, Anticholinergic side effects, Hypotension		If EPS is presented, add benztropine 0.5–1 mg or diphenhydramine 25–50 mg
	If increased sedation desired, add lorazepam 0.5–2 mg				

Figure 4.1 Algorithm for Medicating Agitation. Discussion of each medication is provided in Table 4.2.

Table 4.2 Psychopharmacological Management

haloperidol (Haldol®)—neuroleptic agent potent dopamine blocker; **drug of choice**; effective in diminishing agitation, paranoia and fear	Check vital signs and obtain an EKG. Monitor QTc regularly. Start with low doses (0.5 mg–2 mg dose IV, and double the dose every 30 to 60 minutes until agitation is decreased). Parenteral doses are approximately twice as potent as oral doses.
lorazepam (Ativan®)—should not be given alone when delirium causes agitation, since it may increase confusion	Common strategy is to add parenteral lorazepam (0.5–2 mg IV) to a regimen of haloperidol, which may help to rapidly sedate the agitated delirious patient.
chlorpromazine (Thorazine®)—for a very agitated or combative patient who does not respond	Intravenously (see Figure 4.1), but be alert to potential hypotensive and anticholinergic side effects.
Newer atypical neuroleptic drugs have fewer risks of dystonia, Parkinsonism, and restlessness, but may cause postural hypotension and sedation. In the long term, these medications can cause metabolic syndromes and increased glucose. • olanzapine (Zyprexa®, Zydis®) • risperidone (Risperdal®) • quetiapine (Seroquel®) • ziprasidone (Geodon®)	Elderly or frail patients require lower doses of these medications. Added risks of sedation and postural hypotension in older patients with dementia. May be given intramuscularly. Olanzapine is available in orally disintegrating tablets (Zydis®) and intramuscularly. Risperidone (Risperdal®) is available in orally disintegrating tablets and liquid, if the patient will take oral medications without biting or aggressiveness. These medications can be immediately calming. Elderly patients with dementia related psychosis are at increased risk of death with atypical antipsychotics. Monitor QTc regularly.

Management of Refusal of Treatment or Demand to Leave

Another frequent emergency is the older patient who wants to leave the hospital against medical advice or refuses to accept a discharge disposition to a different living situation (i.e., nursing home, assisted living, or hospice). They might also refuse medical or surgical procedures (i.e., lumbar punctures, placement of central catheters). The oncologist may have to evaluate the patient's capacity to make decisions about medical care. Family and multidisciplinary meetings that include input from family or designated HCPs, occupation and physical therapy, hospital administrators or patient representatives, language interpreters if needed, chaplaincy if appropriate, social work, and the oncology team are recommended (Box 4.3).

Table 4.3 Questions to Ask Patients or Family When Assessing Suicidal Risk

Acknowledge that these are common thoughts that can be discussed	• Older patients with cancer often have had passing thoughts about suicide or death, such as "Maybe it'd be easier for everyone if I weren't alive anymore" or "I might do something if it gets bad enough." Have you ever had thoughts like that?
	• Have you had any thoughts of not wanting to live?
	• Have you had those thoughts in the past few days?
Assess Level of Risk	• Do you have thoughts about wanting to die or end your life? How?
	• Do you have a plan?
	• Do you have any strong social supports?
	• Do you have pills stockpiled at home?
	• Do you own or have access to a weapon?
Obtain Prior History	• Have you ever had a psychiatric disorder, suffered from depression, or made a suicide attempt?
	• Is there a family history of suicide? Do you know anyone who has committed suicide? How did you feel about that?
Identify Substance Abuse	• Have you had a problem with alcohol or drugs?
Identify Bereavement	• Have you lost anyone close to you recently?
Identify Medical Predictors of Risk	• Do you have pain, fatigue or other physical symptoms that are not being relieved that make it difficult to for you to enjoy living?
	• How has the disease affected your life?
	• How is your memory and concentration?
	• Do you feel hopeless?
	• What do you plan for the future?

Table 4.4 Interventions for Suicidal Patient

For patient whose suicidal threat is seen as serious	• Provide constant observation and further assessment.
	• Dangerous objects like guns or intoxicants should be removed from the room or home.
	• The risk for suicidal behavior should be communicated to family members. Some states require registry notification of patients deemed to have a high likelihood of hurting themselves or others.
For patient who is not deemed acutely suicidal and is medically stabilized	• Review with the patient actions s/he can take if feeling overwhelmed or suicidal; consider making a contract with the physician to talk about suicidal thoughts in the future rather than to act on them, and to call for help if needed.
For inpatients	• Room searches should be carried out to make sure there are no means available for self-destructive behavior.
	• The patient should be under constant observation from the time suicidal thoughts are expressed.

(continued)

Table 4.4 (Continued)

For severely suicidal outpatients whose suicidal thoughts are not acutely caused by their medical condition or medication	• Psychiatric hospitalization is warranted, either by voluntary or involuntary means. If suicidal ideation is not related to medical condition or medication, very medically ill patients may not be appropriate admissions to psychiatric units—they may be better treated with 1:1 constant observation on a medical floor. A psychiatrist can assist in making these arrangements. Document medical action and reasoning in the crisis.

Box 4.3 Interventions to Evaluate Treatment Refusal

- Sit down with the patient to find out what he understands about his predicament.
- Do a mental status examination and determine if there is compromise of cognition.
- Until the patient's cognition and judgment are assessed, he can be detained.
- Assess judgment and insight in relation to the specific decision about the procedure or situation.
- Ask, "Does the patient have the capacity (understanding) to make a decision about refusing this MRI scan, or lumbar puncture?"
- The patient may be able to understand the issues related to some decisions and not to others, even in the presence of cognitive compromise or psychosis.
- Family/interdisciplinary meeting to understand changes from baseline medical, physical and psychiatric functioning and gather available supports
- The gravity of the decision to refuse treatment, the life-threatening nature or potential benefit of a decision, guides the depth of the evaluation of a patient's understanding of the illness, treatment recommendations, and consequences of refusing. In complex situations, a psychiatric consultation or an ethics committee review may be helpful.

References

1. Antai-Otong D. Managing geriatric psychiatric emergencies: delirium and dementia. *Nurs Clin N Am*. 2003;38(1):123–135.

2. Borja B, Borja CS, Gade S. Psychiatric emergencies in the geriatric population. Clin Geriatr Med. 2007; 23(2):391–400.

3. Riba, MB, Ravindranath, D., eds. *Clinical Manual of Emergency Psychiatry*. Washington, DC: American Psychiatric Publishing; 2010.

4. Jamshed N, Dubin J, Eldadah Z. Emergency management of palpitations in the elderly: epidemiology, diagnostic approaches, and therapeutic options. *Clin Geriatr Med*. 2013;29(1):205–230.

5. Piechniczek-Buczek J. Psychiatric emergencies in the elderly population. *Emerg Med Clin N Am.* 2006;24(2):467–490.

6. Roth AJ, Breitbart W. Psychiatric emergencies in terminally ill cancer patients. *Hematol/Oncol Clinics of North America.*1996;10, 235–259.

7. Talbot-Stern, Green T, Royle TJ. Psychiatric manifestations of systemic illness. *Emerg Med Clin N Am.* 2000;18(2):199–209.

8. Testa A, Giannuzzi R, Sollazzo F, Petrongolo L, Bernardini L, Daini S. Psychiatric emergencies (part I): psychiatric disorders causing organic symptoms. *Eur Rev Med Pharmacol Sci.* 2013;17(Suppl 1):55–64.

9. Tousi B. Movement disorder emergencies in the elderly: recognizing and treating an often-iatrogenic problem. *Cleve Clin J Med.* 2008;75(6):449–457.

10. Wilhelm S, Schacht A, Wagner T. Use of antipsychotics and benzodiazepines in patients with psychiatric emergencies: results of an observational trial. BMC Psychiatry. 2008; 22(8):61.

11. Zaheer J, Links PS, Liu E. Assessment and emergency management of suicidality in personality disorders. *Psychiatr Clin N Am.* 2008;31(3): viii-ix, 527–543.

Chapter 5

Cognitive Disorders and Delirium

Charissa Andreotti, James C. Root, Yesne Alici, and
Tim A. Ahles

Definitions

Cancer- or cancer-therapy-associated cognitive change refers to disruption in cognitive ability during or following cancer diagnosis and treatment.

Neuropsychological assessment is the formal assessment of cognitive functioning utilizing standardized, validated measures of cognitive ability.

Delirium is an acute change in cognition, behavior, and level of alertness secondary to a general medical condition or medications, and is commonly encountered in hospitalized older adults with cancer.

Non-CNS cancer treatments and therapies are associated with changes in cognitive ability in the elderly. The specific treatments and mechanisms that may affect cognitive abilities remain unclear.[1, for review,2] Evidence has been found for neurotoxic effects of chemotherapy, but these effects do not fully account for all neurophysiological changes and cognitive declines in individuals with cancer. These observations have led to the suggestion that such cognitive changes would be better referred to as "cancer- o cancer-therapy-associated cognitive change" to better address what is likely a multifactorial etiology that may be further complicated by vulnerabilities and comorbidities associated with advanced age. See Boxes 5.1–5.7 and Table 5.1.

Box 5.1 Treatments Impacting Cognition in the Elderly Cancer Patient

- **Systemic chemotherapy treatment.**
- **Endocrine treatment** mainly for breast cancer may include Tamoxifen or aromatase inhibitors for ablation of estrogen.
- **Hormone ablation therapy** for prostate cancer may include centrally acting Leuprolide, Goserelin, or Degarelix or peripherally acting medications like bicalutamide for ablation of testosterone and its function.[3]
- **Surgical resection of primary tumors** as a result of surgical stress, inflammation, anesthetic exposure, and following postoperative delirium.
- **Radiation therapy.**

Box 5.2 Increased Risk for Cognitive Difficulties in the Elderly Cancer Patient

- Older patients present with accumulating comorbidities and potentially diminished functional independence, collectively referred to as "frailty."
- Decreased resistance to stress may also amplify the impairing effects of cancer treatment on the brain and cognition.
- Age-related comorbidities that may increase risk for cognitive decline include:
  - Cardiovascular disease.
  - Hypertension.
  - Diabetes.
- Patients may display age-related neurocognitive changes (e.g., mild cognitive impairment or dementia) prior to undergoing treatment. It is likely that patients with preexisting cognitive vulnerabilities may be especially predisposed to cognitive impairment associated with cancer treatment.

Adapted from Ahles TA, et al. Longitudinal assessment of cognitive changes associated with adjuvant treatment for breast cancer: impact of age and cognitive reserve. *J Clin Oncol.* 2012;28:4434–4440.

Box 5.3 Cognitive Abilities Affected in the Elderly Cancer Patient

Presentation of cognitive difficulties can be variable but may include:

- **Attentional function**—distractibility, difficulties in multi-tasking, and difficulties in sustained concentration.
- **Psychomotor speed**—less-efficient performance of cognitive tasks and feelings of mental slowing.
- **Learning and memory**—difficulties in acquisition of new information and poor recall of newly learned information.
- **Cognitive flexibility**—decreased ability to deal with novel situations or in problem solving.
- **Word finding**—difficulties in accessing words for familiar objects.

Box 5.4 Prevalence of Cognitive Difficulties in the Elderly Cancer Patient

- During active treatment, subject reports of cognitive dysfunction are common (50%) and decrease once treatment is completed.
- Studies on survivors suggest that only a subset of individuals go on to experience and exhibit cognitive dysfunction.
- Objective cognitive dysfunction following completion of treatment, as measured by objective neuropsychological measures, ranges 17 to 75 percent.

Box 5.5 Course of Cognitive Difficulties in the Elderly Cancer Patient

- A subset of individuals diagnosed with cancer exhibit objective cognitive difficulties before treatment.
- Cognitive dysfunction is frequently reported during active treatment.
- A subset of survivors first exhibit cognitive difficulties in the first few months to several years following completion of treatment and may be a result of patients' attempts to return to work or other responsibilities which present increased environmental demands.
- New onset, late effects may also be exhibited.
- The course of cognitive difficulties following treatment is variable, with a subset of survivors experiencing persistent dysfunction up to five years posttreatment completion.
- Still being investigated is whether older cancer survivors may exhibit a steeper decline in cognitive functioning over time following treatment due to potentially accelerated aging initiated by cancer and cancer treatment.

Box 5.6 Ruling Out other Etiologies

- For a subset of elderly cancer patients, cognitive decline following treatment may represent age-appropriate cognitive changes or the beginning of a degenerative dementing condition unrelated to cancer treatment.
- Reversible factors that should be considered in geriatric patients reporting cognitive decline in the context of a cancer diagnosis and treatment include:
  - Substance abuse.
  - Longstanding alcohol use.
  - Vitamin deficiency.
  - Thyroid dysfunction.
- Several common comorbidities in geriatric patients may have a significant impact on cognition:
  - Diabetes.
  - Vascular disease.
  - Epilepsy.
- Medications often used to manage comorbidities or symptoms in geriatric patients (e.g., pain medications, anticholinergic medications) and cases of medication interactions and polypharmacy may contribute to symptoms of cognitive impairment.

Box 5.7 Assessment of Cognitive Functions in the Elderly Cancer Patient

Several brief screening tools for orientation, mental status, and basic cognitive function are available and can be easily administered in both inpatient and outpatient settings, but they lack sensitivity to detect subtle cognitive changes. Patients may benefit from a referral for more extensive neuropsychological evaluation to clarify a diagnosis of cancer-related neurocognitive dysfunction and rule out an incipient dementia.

- Neuropsychological evaluations draw on a collection of standardized paper and pencil and computerized tasks to assess a patient's performance across several cognitive domains, such as verbal and nonverbal reasoning and memory, speed of mental processing, working memory, attention, language, executive function.[5]

- The tasks are normed against population-based means, often stratified by sex, age, ethnicity, and education. As such, a score in the "normal" or "average" range may not signify a lack of impairment, as the patient may have performed in the "above average" range prior to treatment.

- Validated tests of a patient's estimated level of premorbid function can be used to illuminate changes in ability when pretreatment neuropsychological testing results are not available.

- A referral for a comprehensive evaluation of this nature may provide validation of the patient's complaints. In addition, the results obtained may aid in determining the patient's ability to hold employment and any necessary accommodations and can be used for determining the patient's competence to live alone, carry out activities of daily living, and maintain his/her own finances.

Box 5.8 Treatment of Cognitive Dysfunction

- Once a diagnosis of cancer-related or cancer treatment-related cognitive decline has been established, the patient and his/her care-giving team may benefit from cognitive, behavioral, and/or psychopharmacological intervention strategies.
- Cognitive rehabilitation
  - Direct remediation aims to strengthen and restore function to affected cognitive abilities through cognitive drills, although studies demonstrating efficacy are lacking at this time.
  - Cognitive behaviorally oriented therapy may improve coping skills and verbal working memory.
  - Compensatory remediation offers strategies and aides to decrease the effect of cognitive dysfunction on daily life.
    - Calendars.
    - Planners.
    - Timers.
    - Smart-phone applications in order to remind a patient about upcoming appointments and tasks to be completed.

(continued)

Box 5.8 (Continued)

- Behavioral Interventions.
  - Yoga.
  - Exercise.
  - Mindfulness/meditation.
- Psychopharmacological intervention.
  - Methylphenidate and modafinil have been used for cognitive dysfunction, fatigue, and anergia with mixed results.[6]
    - Randomized, double-blind controlled trials with methylphenidate have failed to show a significant evidence of superiority when compared to placebo in adult patients.
    - The studies on modafinil have shown mixed results.
    - Studies with larger sample size and improved study design are needed to better assess the efficacy of pharmacologic interventions in cancer- and cancer-therapy-related cognitive changes.

Box 5.9 Delirium in the Elderly Cancer Patient

- Delirium is an acute change in cognition, behavior, and level of alertness secondary to a general medical condition or medications, and is commonly encountered in hospitalized older adults with cancer.[7] A myriad of cognitive changes can be observed during an episode of delirium:
  - Inattention.
  - Language disturbances.
  - Disorientation.
  - Executive dysfunction.
  - Short term memory impairment.
  - Visuospatial dysfunction.[6]
- About 20–40 percent of hospitalized older adults, and up to 85 percent of patients with advanced cancer develop delirium.[8]
- Risk factors include:
  - Advanced age.
  - Medical comorbidities.
  - Increased falls.
  - Decreased functional independence.
  - Baseline cognitive dysfunction.
- The main differences between delirium and cancer-related or cancer-therapy-associated cognitive changes are the acute onset, fluctuating course of arousal levels, and accompanying behavioral changes that are a part of the delirium phenomenology.
- Long-term effects of delirium include:
  - Significant morbidity and mortality.
  - Long-term cognitive impairment.

(continued)

Box 5.8 (Continued)

- It is important for psycho-oncologists to assess for delirium in hospitalized older adults, to inquire about a history of delirium or pre-existing cognitive deficits among older cancer patients, and to anticipate a higher risk of delirium among patients with cancer-related or cancer-therapy-associated cognitive changes.

- In determining the appropriateness of imaging studies, clinicians should consider several disease-related factors. For example, a change in cognitive function may be an early sign of recurrence in patients with a history of brain tumors. In addition, patients with specific cancer types that have high rates of brain metastases (e.g., lung) may benefit from imaging studies to rule out metastatic disease as an underlying cause of cognitive changes. In patients with other cancer diagnoses (e.g., early stage breast cancer) who report cognitive changes, an imaging referral may not be justified in the absence of other neurologic findings such as headache, lateralized weakness, or sensory changes.

Table 5.1 Neurocognitive Measures, Screening Measures, and Delirium Assessments

Measure	Function
Premorbid Intelligence	
Test of Premorbid Functioning (TOPF)	A measure estimating premorbid cognitive abilities, correlated with general intellectual abilities
Verbal Ability	
FAS-Controlled Oral Word Association Test (FAS-COWAT)	A timed measure of phonemic fluency
Animal Naming Test	A timed measure of semantic fluency
Boston Naming Test (BNT)	A measure of confrontation naming (word finding)
Learning and Memory	
California Verbal Learning Test II (CVLT-II)	A measure of word list learning and recall
Hopkins Verbal Learning Test— Revised (HVLT-R)	A measure of word list learning and recall
Logical Memory I and II (WMS-IV)	A measure of verbal story learning and recall
Rey-Osterreith Complex Figure	A measure of visual figure learning and recall
Brief Visuospatial Memory Test— Revised (BVMT-R)	A measure of visual figure learning and recall
Attention	
Digit Span (WAIS-IV)	A measure of brief span of attention
Arithmetic (WAIS-IV)	A measure of brief span of attention and working memory
Continuous Performance Test (CPT)	A measure of sustained attention

(continued)

Table 5.1 (Continued)

Measure	Function
Psychomotor Speed	
The Trail Making Test (Part A)	A speeded grapho-motor measure of visual scanning
The Trail Making Test (Part B)	A speeded grapho-motor measure, visual scanning, and set-shifting
Digit Symbol—Coding (WAIS-IV)	A speeded graphomotor measure
Symbol Search (WAIS-IV)	A speeded measure of visual scanning attention
Motor Speed and Dexterity	
Finger Tapping Test	A speeded measure of manual dexterity
Grooved Pegboard	A speeded measure of fine motor dexterity
Visual Reasoning/Construction	
Rey-Osterreith Complex Figure	A measure of visual construction
Judgment of Line Orientation	A measure of visuospatial judgment and reasoning
Block Design (WAIS-IV)	A timed measure of visual construction and reasoning
Executive Functioning	
Wisconsin Card Sorting Task (WCST)	A measure of abstract reasoning and problem solving
Stroop	A measure of word reading, color naming, and inhibition
Tower of London[†]	A measure of planning and problem solving
Psychological/Emotional	
Personality Assessment Inventory (PAI)	A self-report measure of psychological functioning
Beck Depression Inventory (BDI)	A self-report measure of depressive symptoms
State Trait Anxiety Inventory (STAI)	A self-report measure of anxiety symptoms
Mental Status	
Mini-Mental State Exam (MMSE)	A brief measure of mental status
Short Test of Mental Status (STMS)	A brief measure of mental status
Mini-Cog	A brief measure of executive function and word registration/recall
Delirium Assessments	
Confusion Assessment Method (CAM)	Clinician administered measure of delirium
Confusion Assessment Method (CAM)—ICU Version	Clinician administered measure of delirium for use with mechanically ventilated patients.
Memorial Delirium Assessment Scale (MDAS)	Clinician administered measure of delirium

References

1. Ahles TA, Saykin AJ. Candidate mechanisms for chemotherapy-induced cognitive changes. *Nat Rev Cancer.* 2007;7:192–201.

2. Ahles TA, Root JC, Ryan, EL. Cancer- and cancer treatment-associated cognitive change: an update on the state of the science. *J Clin Oncol.* 2012;30:3675–3686. doi:10.1200/JCO.2012.43.0116

3. Nelson CJ, Lee JS, Gamboa MC, Roth AJ. Cognitive effects of hormone therapy in men with prostate cancer: a review. *Cancer.* 2008;113:1097–1106. doi:10.1002/cncr.23658 (2008).

4. Ahles TA, et al. Longitudinal assessment of cognitive changes associated with adjuvant treatment for breast cancer: impact of age and cognitive reserve. *J Clin Oncol.* 2010;28:4434–4440. doi:10.1200/JCO.2009.27.0827

5. Strauss E, Sherman, EMS, Spreen, O. *A Compendium of Neuropsychological Tests: Administration, Norms, and Commentary,* 3rd ed. New York, NY: Oxford University Press; 2006.

6. Von Ah D, Storey S, Jansen CE, Allen DH. Coping strategies and interventions for cognitive changes in patients with cancer. *Sem Oncol Nurs.* 2013;29:288–299, doi:10.1016/j.soncn.2013.08.009

7. Breitbart W, Alici Y. Agitation and delirium at the end of life: "We couldn't manage him." *JAMA.* 2008;300:2898–2910, E2891. doi:10.1001/jama.2008.885

8. Breitbart W, Alici Y. Evidence-based treatment of delirium in patients with cancer. *J Clin Oncol.* 2012;30:1206–1214. doi:10.1200/JCO.2011.39.8784

Chapter 6

Depressive Spectrum Disorders and Grief

Andrew J. Roth, Mindy Greenstein, Talia Weiss Wiesel, and
Steven Schulberg

Introduction

Depression is characterized by feeling sad, hopeless, and/or
discouraged.[1] These feelings may be accompanied by irritability, loss
of pleasure, reduced concentration, and physical symptoms such as
changes in appetite and sleep patterns, psychomotor disturbance, gastric upset, nausea, or nonspecific complaints of body aches or pains,
and fatigue. In the elderly, somatic symptoms of depression may be
more prominent than in younger people. Levels of depressed symptoms
in the context of cancer vary from sadness to true major depression,
usually mixed with anxiety, and often focused on helplessness related
to illness. Physical or neurovegetative symptoms may be more related
to cancer or cancer treatment than to depression, though loved ones
may think the patient is depressed as is common with physically healthy
people. Mood disorder (depression) due to general medical condition
is common in medically compromised patients whose symptoms of
depression can be linked to their medical situation. Preexisting depressive disorders may complicate care.

Older patients, although representing a large and growing proportion of
those with cancer, have systematically been underrepresented in research
studies.[2] Depression in these older adults ranges from 17 to 26 percent.[3,4]
The presentation of depression in the elderly frequently appears as minor
or subsyndromal depression, or an adjustment disorder, that is due to a
recent challenging situation, with an estimated rate of 15–25 percent in
medically ill patients.[5] Kua suggests that as many as a third of elderly cancer
patients may experience some form of psychological distress.[6] Additionally,
older age is a risk factor for suicide in cancer patients.[7]

Understanding the unique nuances and relationships of depression,
cancer, and older age is key to improved diagnosis and treatment, and
ultimately better quality of life and adherence to cancer treatment
regimens.

Underdiagnosis and Undertreatment of Depression in the Elderly

Although several studies have reported lower rates of depressive disorders in elderly cancer patients compared to younger ones, this may be because rates of depression are underestimated.[8] See Boxes 6.1 and 6.2 for the reasons for underdiagnosis of depression and common symptoms of major depression in older adults with cancer.

Box 6.1 Reasons for Underdiagnosis of Depression in the Elderly

1. Older patients do not readily complain of mental symptoms.
2. Older patients are more likely to present with somatic symptoms of depression, rather than psychological ones.
3. Physicians dismiss distress symptoms as due to "old age" (ageism).
4. Common depression diagnostic scales are not sensitive or specific to older people with cancer.
5. Physical symptoms of depression can overlap with—or be misattributed to—the cancer or treatment side effects and vice versa.

Box 6.2 Common Symptoms of Major Depression in Older Adults with Cancer

- *Depressed or irritable mood most of the day, most days,* for at least 2 weeks.
- *Decreased interest or pleasure in most activities, not due to physical. Symptoms of cancer (i.e., pain or fatigue), its treatment or other medical conditions or treatment.*
- *Somatic complaints such as achiness, gastric upset, headaches, and joint pain may be important indicators of depression in older patients (these may be difficult to distinguish from cancer- or aging-related problems; these can cause depression, or be symptoms of it).*
- *Feelings of worthlessness (i.e., feeling like a burden) or excessive, inappropriate guilt.*
- *Suicidality: Thoughts of death or suicide, or having a suicide plan* (ideations about dying are common in older people with cancer). Having intent or an active plan to hurt oneself is an indicator of acuity.
- Change in appetite or weight not related to cancer or its treatment.
- Change in sleep: Insomnia or hypersomnia not related to cancer or its treatment.
- Change in activity: Psychomotor agitation or retardation not related to cancer or its treatment.
- Fatigue or loss of energy not related to cancer or its treatment.
- Concentration: decreased ability to think or concentrate, or more indecisiveness.

Box 6.3 Periods of Increased Vulnerability for the Elderly Patient with Cancer

- Finding a suspicious physical symptom.
- Hardship of medical work-up.
- Waiting for biopsy results.
- Finding out the cancer diagnosis.
- Treatment decisions: Should I treat the cancer or not (at my age): if yes, which treatment will have the best results with the least compromise to my quality of life.
- Awaiting treatment.
- Conclusion of treatment regiments (successful or not).
- Stopping ineffective treatment regimens and decisions to move to others.

Endicott has recommended that the neurovegetative symptoms of depression be substituted with psychological symptoms: Physical/somatic symptoms (change in appetite/weight; sleep disturbance; fatigue, loss of energy; diminished ability to think or concentrate) are replaced by psychological symptoms (tearfulness, depressed appearance; social withdrawal, decreased talkativeness; brooding, self-pity, pessimism; lack of reactivity, blunting).[9] It is not clear how helpful this approach is in the elderly given the prominence of somatic symptoms as common identifiers of depression.

Periods of Increased Vulnerability

Periods of increased vulnerability in older adults with cancer are outlined in Box 6.3.[10]

Risk Factors for Depression

Risk Factors for Depression are outlined in Box 6.4.

Box 6.4 Risk Factors for Depression

A. Physical/Treatment-Related Risk Factors
   1. Uncontrolled pain.
   2. Decline in health/increase in disability.
   3. Sensory losses (hearing, vision, ambulatory).
   4. Increased age.[11]
   5. Fatigue.
   6. Physical and cognitive decline.

(continued)

Box 6.4 (Continued)

7. Polypharmacy.

8. Certain anticancer drugs (e.g., corticosteroids).

9. Certain cancer types: pancreatic, head and neck, and lung cancers.

10. Somatic complaints of achiness, gastric upset, headaches, joint pain (which can cause depression, or be symptoms of it).

B. Emotional/Social Risk Factors for Depression in the Elderly

1. Lack of perceived control.

2. Other life stresses or losses.

3. Loneliness or feeling isolated.

4. Fatalistic feelings.

5. Inadequacy of emotional support.

6. *Grief: Loss of spouse and others in social network.

7. Obituary Observations/Surveillance.

8. Dwindling financial resources.

9. Unmet need for practical assistance.

10. Women are at higher risk than men.

11. African American (as opposed to Caucasians).[12]

12. Lower level education

13. History of emotional problems

14. Family history of depression or suicide

* Grief is a normal reaction to a major loss. Sometimes symptoms of grief overlap with major depression. The recent edition of DSM -513 no longer excludes from a major depressive disorder diagnosis depressive symptoms lasting fewer than 2 months following the death of a loved one. On the one hand, this may increasingly pathologize grief reactions, causing more people to be treated with pharmacologic agents. On the other hand, it may cue practitioners to take more seriously the severe suffering of someone who is having a depressive disorder over and above his or her bereavement.

Negative Sequelae of Depression

Negative sequelae of depression are outlined in Box 6.5.

Identifying Risk Factors for Suicide and Suicidal Ideation

Older patients with cancer are at increased risk of developing suicidal ideation compared to the population at large.[18] Furthermore, the actual suicide completion rates are on average 50 percent higher in cancer patients than in a medically healthy population.[19,20]

It is important to identify patients at higher relative suicide risk who have an immediate plan of action as well as intent to carry it out. A history of prior suicide attempts or a history of depression, anxiety, or other mental illness or psychiatric hospitalization increases their risk. Often patients who have a desire for hastened death and passive thoughts that life is not

Box 6.5 Negative Sequelae of Depression

- Decreased adherence to treatment regimens and longer hospital stays.[14]
- Physiologic changes associated with depression, such as fatigue, poor appetite, and decreased motivation, can increase risk factors for developing new medical diseases and can worsen the course and treatment outcome of an already established medical illness.[15]
- Interference with the ability to make treatment decisions and adhere to lengthy treatment.[16] (Katon W, Lin, & Kroenke, 2007).
- Poor quality of life
- Increased loneliness
- Increased frustration/irritability (lower tolerance)
- If depression is accompanied by cognitive deficits, it may be harbinger of cognitive disorder or dementia
- Suicide.[17] (Rao A & Cohen HJ, 2004).

Box 6.6 Recognizing patients at higher risk for suicide

- Tumor staging and metastases at diagnoses are red flags for higher suicide risk.[18,23]
- Poor prognosis and advanced staging at diagnosis.[18,19,24]
- Tumor site: lung and other respiratory cancers usually have the highest suicide rates for both men and women. Other sites associated with higher risk are head and neck, stomach, pancreas, and colon.[18,19,25]
- Cancers that can lead to deforming surgeries.
- Time since diagnosis: 1/3 of cancer related suicides occur within the first month.[26] Rates remain high for the first six months.
- Patients with a history of depression, or who openly express feelings of hopelessness and being a burden.[27]
- Severe pain that is constant and poorly controlled [7,25,28]

worth living anymore, can still be future oriented and hopeful about some aspects of their lives, therefore lowering their risk.[21]

Suicidal ideation screening is an important tool for evaluating older patients with cancer. Asking about suicide will not put the idea into a patient's head, though asking may serve to legitimize their concerns and give hope that they can be addressed.[21,22] Recruiting a psychosocial support system for the patient can be helpful. It is also essential to treat any underlying conditions that compromise quality of life, such as pain, fatigue, depression, and anxiety, as they may exacerbate the patient's suicidal thoughts and poor outlook.

If a medically ill inpatient has a high suicide risk, he or she should immediately be placed under one-to-one supervision in his or her hospital room, having removed potentially harmful devices, such as medications or sharp objects. These steps will help prevent self-harm. Box 6.6 outlines risk factors for suicide in this population. The NCCN has developed guidelines for identifying and treating depression in cancer patients. Considerations should be given for appropriate alterations in older cancer patients. See Figures 6.1a and b.

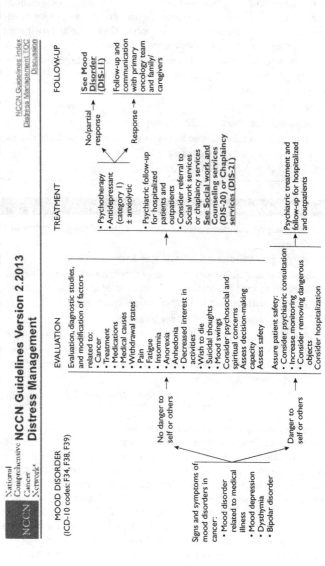

Figure 6.1 NCCN Distress Management Guideline DIS-10, DIS-11—Mood Disorder. Adapted from *Holland JC, Andersen B, Breitbart WS, et al. Distress management. J NCCN Cancer 1 2013;11(2):190–209*

National Comprehensive **NCCN Guidelines Version 2.2013**
NCCN Cancer Network®
Distress Management

NCCN Guidelines Index
Distress Management TOC
Discussion

MOOD DISORDER (continued)
(ICD-10 codes: F34, F38, F39)

EVALUATION   TREATMENT   FOLLOW-UP

No or partial response to treatment for signs and symptoms of mood disorder in cancer → Reevaluate diagnosis and response/adjust medications as indicated ± psychotherapy

No/partial response

Response

• Consider augmenting or changing medications
• Consider electroconvulsive therapy
• Consider consult/second opinion

→ Follow-up and communication with primary oncology team and family/caregivers

Figure 6.1 (Continued)

CHAPTER 6 **Depressive Spectrum Disorders**

65

Medication Options to Treat Depression in Older Cancer Patients

Table 6.1 outlines medication and dosages to treat depression in older cancer patients.

Table 6.1 Medication Options to Treat Depression in Older Cancer Patients		
Medication	**Starting Daily Dose (mg PO)**	**Comments**
Serotonin Reuptake Inhibitors (SSRIs)		
Citalopram	10	SSRI's are generally well tolerated in the older cancer patient. They may increase energy but may extend to anxiety and insomnia. They may be calming but extend to daytime sleepiness; Other side effects include gastric upset and sexual dysfunction.
Escitalopram	5	
Fluoxetine	10	
Paroxetine	10	
Sertraline	25	
Serotonin-Norepinephrine (SNRIs)		
Duloxetine	20	SNRIs have similar side effect profiles as SSRI's. They are also used to treat neuropathic pain syndromes.
Venlafaxine	25	
Others		
Bupropion	100 Slow Release	Bupropion is energizing and can help fatigue. It is contraindicated in people with seizure history or bulimia; it does not cause sexual dysfunction; it is also used as a smoking cessation aide.
Mirtazapine	15–30	Mirtazapine has no gastric side effects and may improve appetite and cause weight gain. It can be sedating and aid sleep.
Psychostimulants		
Dextroamphetamine	2.5	Modafinil and Armodafinil are gentler and more easily tolerated stimulants than the others. It is safer in those with a history of seizures or cardiac arrhythmias.
Methylphenidate	(at 8am & 1pm)	
Modafinil/Armodafinil	2.5 (at 8am & 1pm) 50 (in the morning)	
See Chapter 3, Psychosocial Interventions for Older Cancer Patients.		

Summary

Depression in older cancer patients can be a diagnostic dilemma and can lead to underdiagnosis and undertreatment. Symptomatology differs from younger, healthier adults. Oncology clinicians should be aware of coexisting medical issues and patient frailty when trying to assess and treat depression. Given the prevalence of suicide in older cancer patients, clinicians should be vigilant about screening this population for these symptoms.

References

1. American Psychiatric Association. *Diagnostic and Statistical Manual of mental Disorders* (Fourth Edition, Text Revision ed.). Washington DC: Author; 2000.

2. Aapro M, Extermann M, Repetto L. (2000). Evaluation of the elderly with cancer. *Ann Oncol.* 2000;11(Suppl 3):223–229.

3. Yesne Alici, Talia Weiss, Jimmie C. Holluand, Christian Nelson, Andrew Roth. Common psychiatric problems in older patients with cancer: Report of one-year experience of a psychiatry outpatient clinic. Journal of Geriatric Oncology, Vol. 2, Isse 2, p137–141.

4. Kurtz M, Kurtz J, Stommel M, Given C, Given B. Physical functioning and depression among older persons with cancer. *Cancer Practice.* 2001;9:11–18.

5. Lyness JM. (2004). Treatment of depressive conditions in later life: real-world light for dark (or dim) tunnels. *JAMA.* 2004 291: 1626–1628.

6. Kua J. The prevalence of psychological and psychiatric sequelae of cancer in the elderly: How much do we know? *Ann Acc Med Singapore.* 2005;34:250–256.

7. Walker J., Waters R. A., Murray G, et al. Better off dead: suicidal thoughts in cancer patients. *J Clin Oncol.* 2008;26(29):4725–4730.

8. Weinberger M, Bruce M, Roth A, Breitbart W, Nelson C. (2011). Depression and barriers to mental health care in older cancer patients. *Internl J Geriatr Psychiat.* 2011;26(1):21–26.

9. Endicott J. Measurement of depression in patients with cancer. *Cancer.* 1984;53(Suppl 10):2243–2249.

10. NCCN. Distress management. In: *The Complete Library of NCCN Clinical Practice Guidelines in Oncology.* Jenkintown, PA: National Comprehensive Cancer Network; 2008.

11. Nelson CJ, Balk EM, Roth AJ. Distress, anxiety, depression, and emotional well-being in African-American men with prostate cancer. Psycho-Oncol. 2010;19:1052–1060.

12. Kurtz M, Kurtz J, Stommel M, Given C, Given B. Predictors of depressive symptomatology of geriatric patients with colorectal cancer. *Support Care in Cancer.* 2002;10:494–501.

13. American Psychiatric Association. Diagnostic and Statistical Manual of Mental Disorders 5th ed. Arlington, VA: American Psychiatric Publishing; 2013.

14. Miller K, Massie MJ. (2010). Depressive disorders. In Holland J, Breitbart W, Jacobsen PB, Lederberg M, Loscalzo M & McCorkle R, eds., *Psycho-Oncology.* 2nd ed. New York: Oxford University Press; 2010: 311–318.

15. Roth AJ, Modi R. Psychiatric issues in older cancer patients. *Critical reviews in oncology/hematology*. 2003;48:185–197.

16. Katon W, Lin E., Kroenke K. (2007). The association of depression and anxiety with medical symptom burden in patients with chronic medical illness. *Gen Hosp Psychiat*. 2007; 29:147–155.

17. Rao A, Cohen HJ. Symptom management in the elderly cancer patient: fatigue, pain, and depression. *J Natl Cancer Inst*. 2004;32:150–157.

18. Misono S, Weiss NS, Fann JR, Redman M, Yueh B. Incidence of suicide in persons with cancer. *J Clin Oncol*. 2008;26(29):4731–4738.

19. Dormer N, McCaul K, Kristjanson L. Risk of suicide in cancer patients in western australia, 1981–2002. *Med J Aust*. 2008;188(3):140–143.

20. Yousaf U, Christensen M, Engholm G, Storm HH. Suicides among Danish cancer patients 1971-1999. *Br J Cancer*. 2005;92(6):995–1000.

21. Roth AJ, Weiss TR. Psychiatric emergencies. In: Holland JC, Breitbart WS, Jacobsen PB, Lederberg MS, Loscalzo MJ, McCorkle R, eds. *Psycho-oncology*. 2nd ed. New York, NY: Oxford University Press; 2010:297–302.

22. Massie MJ, Gagnon P, Holland JC. Depression and suicide in patients with cancer. *J Pain Sympt Manage*. 1994;9(5):325–340.

23. Carlsson S, Sandin F, Fall K, et al. Risk of suicide in men with low-risk prostate cancer. *Eur J Cancer*. 2013;49(7):1588–1599.

24. Hem E, Loge JH, Haldorsen T, Ekeberg Ø. Suicide risk in cancer patients from 1960 to 1999. *J Clin Oncol*. 2004;22(20):4209–4216.

25. Akechi T, Nakano T, Akizuki N, et al. Clinical factors associated with suicidality in cancer patients. *Japanese J Clin Oncol*. 2002;32(12):506–511.

26. Johnson TV, Garlow SJ, Brawley OW, Master VA. Peak window of suicides occurs within the first month of diagnosis: Implications for clinical oncology. *Psychooncol*. 2012;21(4):351–356.

27. Schneider KL, Shenassa E. Correlates of suicide ideation in a population-based sample of cancer patients. *J Psychosoc Oncol*. 2008;26(2):49–62.

28. Recklitis CJ, Lockwood RA, Rothwell MA, Diller LR. Suicidal ideation and attempts in adult survivors of childhood cancer. *J Clin Oncol*. 2006;24(24):3852–3857.

Chapter 7

Anxiety Disorders

Tatiana D. Starr, Talia Weiss Wiesel, and Yesne Alici

Introduction

Anxiety, described as excessive worry or fear, manifests itself as a disturbance in mood, thinking, behavior, and physiological activity[1] for old and
young alike. Typical anxiety symptoms that present without illness include
thoughts of impending doom; overgeneneralizing—that is, a cognitive
error wherein a person sees a sole occurrence as an invariable rule—and
catastrophizing—that is, an irrational thought of believing that something
is far worse than it actually is; inability to absorb information; and inability
to adhere to recommended procedures.[2] However, within the context of
cancer, patients may also have anxiety related to fear of death, fears for the
future and family, and loss of control.

Some degree of anxiety is experienced by most cancer patients during their course of illness, often presenting during crisis points such as
initial diagnosis, initiation of treatment, unsuccessful treatment, and cancer recurrence.[2] In the face of a life-threatening illness, anxiety can often
be viewed as an appropriate, expected, and even "normal" reaction to a
stressful and traumatic event. It can, therefore, be difficult to determine
when a patient's anxiety exceeds the typical range, and it should not be
normalized but, rather, should receive specific attention, assessment, and
potential intervention. In general, further evaluation is needed when a
patient's anxiety persists beyond the immediate time frame of a stressor
and causes impairment in overall functioning.[2]

Among older adults with cancer, comorbid medical conditions, frailty,
social isolation, poor social support, and fear of worsening physical and
cognitive functioning may increase vulnerability to anxiety syndromes.

Prevalence

The prevalence of anxiety increases with advancing disease, decline in the
patient's physical status, and worsening frailty. In older cancer patients,
anxiety is commonly associated with depressive symptoms. Anxiety has
been reported in 10 to 28 percent, of advanced cancer patients. Though
prevalence rates of anxiety in the geriatric oncology population are not
well studied, reported rates range from 2.5%–23%.[3] In a recent one-year
survey of 239 elderly cancer patients referred for psychiatric consultation

at the Memorial Sloan Kettering Counseling Center, 5.9 percent were diagnosed with an "other anxiety disorder" and 2.5 percent were diagnosed with an anxiety disorder due to a GMC.[3]

Clinical Features

Anxiety can present with both cognitive and somatic symptoms

Cognitive symptoms may include:[4,5]
- Fear of death.
- Loss of control.
- Feeling of impending doom.
- Overgeneralizing.
- Catastrophizing.

Somatic symptoms may include:[4–6]
- Tachycardia.
- Tachypnea.
- Shortness of breath.
- Diaphoresis.
- Dry mouth.
- Insomnia.
- Gastrointestinal issues.
- Nausea.
- Trembling.
- Tremor.
- Dizziness.

Assessment

A multimodal biopsychosocial assessment is recommended. Consideration of multiple factors including description of the timing of onset of symptoms as well as the quality, frequency, duration and triggers of symptoms, will help the clinician determine the etiology of the anxiety syndrome (preexisting or secondary to cancer diagnosis or treatment) and to create a viable treatment plan.[7]

A comprehensive medical history and physical evaluation is important to assess vital signs as well as cardiovascular, neurological, gastrointestinal, and respiratory systems whose syndromes may mimic or exacerbate anxiety. If the symptoms of anxiety are found to be an exacerbation of a preexisting anxiety disorder in the context of a cancer diagnosis or recurrence,[6] treatment of the primary underlying disorder may be the most effective way to alleviate the symptoms of anxiety. Other patients may develop a new anxiety disorder following their cancer diagnosis.

Anxiety disorders are common in the general population. Anxiety disorders found in the cancer setting include adjustment disorder with anxiety with or without depressive symptoms and anxiety disorder due to a general medical condition (GMC), both of which are directly related to the cancer diagnosis or treatment, as well as preexisting anxiety disorders such as panic disorder, or generalized anxiety disorder, that are exacerbated by the cancer course and can complicate care. Posttraumatic stress disorder can be found in current patients who have experienced a trauma before the cancer (i.e., combat) or de novo in those who feel traumatized by the cancer or treatment (i.e., very painful cancer course, or high dose chemotherapy with extended, complicated hospitalizations in bone marrow transplant patients), or in survivors after their treatment has concluded. Additionally, phobias, such as fear of needles, or claustrophobia may present additional challenges for patients who must undergo multiple tests and procedures such as magnetic resonance imaging, injections, and intravenous treatments. An anxiety response could also be conditioned. For instance, symptoms of restlessness and fear may emerge as an anticipatory response to a repeated aversive treatment like chemotherapy, when the patient approaches the hospital, or as the nurse enters in the chemotherapy suite.[5,10]

Anxiety is often experienced as a reaction to the threat of a potentially life-threatening disease. For these patients, anxiety can increase in the following settings or conditions:[6]

- Initial diagnosis.
- Anticipation of check-ups.
- Diagnostic studies that might detect recurrence and that involve waiting for results.
- Advancing disease.
- Receiving news of poor prognosis.
- Paradoxically, at the end of active treatment.
- When surveillance intervals between visits with the oncology team are increased.

Patients who are successfully treated for their cancer may also experience chronic anxiety associated with fear of recurrence. Additionally, patients who undergo genetic testing may also worry excessively about their health as well as the health of their families.[6]

Diagnosis is often made on the basis of clinical interview, but screening tools can be an effective and efficient way to alert the oncology team to symptoms of anxiety. Screening can be done as a single symptom assessment (e.g., using the distress thermometer,[7,8] or simply asking "Are you worried?" which may be ideal for a busy clinician, but may lack reliability). Clinicians can also use multiple symptom assessments such as the anxiety subscales on the Memorial Symptom Assessment Scale,[11] the Edmonton Symptom Assessment Scale,[12] the Hospital Anxiety and Depression Questionnaire (HADS),[13] the Brief Symptom Inventory,[14] the Spielberger State Trait Anxiety Inventory,[15] or the Generalized Anxiety Disorder-7 (GAD-7).[16] Clinicians can also assess the clinical syndrome (i.e., GAD, panic disorder, or social phobia disorder), as classified by the *Diagnostic and Statistical Manual of Mental Disorders*, 5th ed. (*DSM-5*).[17] See Boxes 7.1, 7.2, and 7.3.

Box 7.1 *DSM-5* Criteria

Summary of the *DSM-5* Criteria for Generalized Anxiety Disorder

1. Excessive anxiety and worry (apprehensive expectation), occurring more days than not for at least 6 months, about a number of issues.
2. The individual finds it difficult to control the worry.
3. The anxiety and worry are associated with three (or more) of the following six symptoms that have been present for more days than not in the last six months.
   - Restlessness or feeling on edge.
   - Being easily fatigued.
   - Difficulty concentrating.
   - Irritability.
   - Muscle tension.
   - Sleep disturbance (difficulty falling or staying asleep, or restless unsatisfying sleep).
4. The anxiety, worry, or physical symptoms cause clinically significant distress or impairment in important areas of functioning.
5. The disturbance is not attributable to the physiological effects of a substance or another medical condition.
6. The disturbance is not better explained by another mental disorder.

Summary of the *DSM-5* Criteria for Anxiety Disorder Due to Another Medical Condition

- Panic attacks or anxiety is predominant in the clinical picture.
- There is evidence from the history, physical examination, or laboratory findings that the disturbance is the direct pathophysiological consequence of another medical condition.
- The disturbance is not better explained by another mental disorder or delirium.
- The disturbance causes clinically significant distress or impairment in important areas of functioning.

Adapted from *Diagnostic and Statistical Manual of Mental Disorders.* 5th ed. Arlington, VA: American Psychiatric Association; 2013.

Differential Diagnosis

Diagnosing anxiety disorders in the elderly is particularly challenging due to the increased likelihood of comorbid medical and psychological conditions and ongoing pharmacologic treatments that may complicate the clinical picture.[18] Patients with the following conditions may appear anxious or may present with anxiety, where the appropriate treatment is to address the underlying physiological cause and to provide education and support:

Box 7.2 Periods of Increased Vulnerability in the Elderly

- Finding a symptom suspicious for cancer recurrence.
- During work-up.
- Finding out the diagnosis.

Transitions in treatment, e.g., awaiting treatment, changes in treatment modality, end of treatment, treatment failure.

- Discharge from hospital after treatment.
- Stresses of survivorship.
- Medical follow-up and surveillance.
- Recurrence.
- Advanced cancer.
- End of life.

Adapted from NCCN. Distress management. *The Complete Library of NCCN Clinical Practice Guidelines in Oncology.* Jenkintown, PA: National Comprehensive Cancer Network; 2008.

Box 7.3 Risk Factors for Anxiety in the Elderly

1. Pain.
2. Functional disability.
3. Need for assistance with activities of daily living.
4. Poor physical condition.
5. Comorbid medical conditions.
6. Poor eyesight.

- Pain and poor symptom control of fatigue, depression, insomnia, dyspnea, and nausea can present with anxiety symptoms.—Patients experiencing these symptoms may appear anxious; however the anxious symptoms often dissipate with adequate treatment.
- Delirium—Patients who are delirious exhibit symptoms associated with anxiety including restlessness, agitation, and impulsivity.
- Hypoxia or respiratory distress—Patients experiencing respiratory distress may also appear to be anxious. This anxiety can exacerbate overlapping symptoms such as increased shortness of breath thus creating more anxiety.
- Pulmonary embolus—Patients experiencing an acute event, such as a pulmonary embolus, may also present as anxiety.
- Sepsis, endocrine abnormalities, hypoglycemia, hypercalcemia, hyperthyroidism, and hormone-secreting tumors may all be associated with symptoms of anxiety.[19]
- Medications—Some medications, such as antiemetics, corticosteroids, or bronchodilators, can cause anxiety or akathisia, and withdrawal from alcohol or benzodiazepines are also associated with symptoms of anxiety.[2]

Management

The primary goals for treating anxiety disorders in older cancer patients include reducing the patient's overall level of distress and specific target symptoms that may impair functioning. It is important to take into consideration the etiology, presentation, and setting of the anxious symptoms. Other considerations include problematic patient behavior such as adherence to treatment as well as family and staff reactions to the patient's distress.

Psychotherapeutic treatment options include psychoeducation and cognitive therapy to address a patient's automatic, yet irrational or unrealistic thoughts that lead to excessive worrying, with a more credible and accurate perspective. Several behavioral approaches may also be effective in reducing symptoms of anxiety and include methods such as progressive muscle relaxation, breathing exercises, meditation, hypnosis, biofeedback, systematic desensitization, distraction, and guided imagery.[9]

Negative Sequelae of Anxiety

- Decreased adherence to treatment regimens and longer hospital stays.[20]
- Poor lifestyle behaviors (i.e., substance or tobacco use) that increase risk factors for developing new medical diseases.[18]
- Interference with the ability to make treatment decisions and adhere to lengthy treatment.[21]
- Suicide.[22]

Psychopharmacological Intervention

The pharmacotherapy of anxiety in older adults with cancer involves the judicious use of antidepressants, benzodiazepines, and antipsychotics. Although clinical evidence supports the use of the medications listed in Table 7.1 in the treatment of anxiety among older adults with cancer, randomized controlled trials are required to establish the risks and benefits of medication use for this patient population. Even milder forms of anxiety require attention. Using medication to treat symptoms of anxiety can be beneficial but should be approached carefully with elderly patients. In younger patients, benzodiazepines may be the first line of treatment; however, with older patients, clinicians may want to try alternative medications first, such as buspirone or an antidepressant, yet consider using lower doses of a benzodiazepine if needed.[2] See Table 7.1. Psychotherapy and Behavioral Interventions can be found in Chapter 10, "Psychosocial Interventions for Elderly Cancer Patients."

Table 7.1 Pharmacological Treatment of Anxiety

Medication	Daily Dosage Range*	Comments
Benzodiazepines All benzodiazepines may cause sedation, falls, confusion, and respiratory depression in older cancer patients.		
Alprazolam	0.125–0.5 mg bid to qid Extended release formulation is for daily dosing	Immediate release is short-acting and may need frequent dosing to avoid rebound anxiety; relatively rapid onset
Lorazepam	0.5–2 mg bid to tid	Available in an IV form; intermediate acting
Diazepam	2–10 mg bid to tid	Available in an IV form
Clonazepam	0.125 mg–1 mg bid to tid	Orally disintegrating tablets are useful for patients who have difficulty swallowing; long-acting
Nonbenzodiazepines		
Buspirone	5–20 mg tid	Can take several weeks to start to see improvement; well tolerated, no withdrawal
Antidepressants (Please refer to chapter 7, section A for a list of antidepressants and dosing)		
SSRIs; SNRIs	Various	Can help prevent anxiety when taken daily; can take several weeks to see improvement
Antipsychotics**		
Haloperidol Olanzapine Quetiapine	0.25–2 mg q 4–12 h 2.5–5 mg at bedtime or q 12 hours 12.5–50 mg daily or bid	Haloperidol is also available in IV formulations. No effect on respiration; less likely to cause confusion than benzodiazepines; all antipsychotics may prolong QT interval to varying degrees

ODT = Orally disintegrating tablet; SSRI = Selective serotonin reuptake inhibitors.

*Smaller daily doses can be considered in older, frail adults to avoid side effects.

** Clinicians should consider the risks and benefits of the use of antipsychotics carefully when treating older adults, especially those with underlying cognitive problems due to reports of increased mortality, increased risk of cardiovascular and cerebrovascular events among older adults with dementia treated with antipsychotics.

Adapted from Winell J, Roth AJ. Psychiatric assessment and symptom management in elderly cancer patients. *Oncol.* Oct 2005;19(11):1479–1490; discussion 1492, 1497, 1501–1477.

References

1. U.S. Department of Health and Human Services. *Mental Health: A Report of the Surgeon General*. Rockville, MD: U.S. Department of Health and Human Services, Substance Abuse and Mental Health Services Administration, Center for Mental Health Services, National Institutes of Health, National Institute of Mental Health;1999.

2. Winell J, Roth AJ. Psychiatric assessment and symptom management in elderly cancer patients. *Oncol*. Oct 2005;19(11):1479–1490; discussion 1492, 1497, 1501–1477.

3. Evcimen Y, Holland J, Roth A, Nelson C, Weiss T. Common psychiatric problems in older patients with cancer: Report of one-year experience of a psychiatry outpatient clinic. *Journal of Geriatric Oncology*. 2011;2(2):137–141.

4. Barraclough J. ABC of palliative care. depression, anxiety, and confusion. BMJ. Nov 22 1997;315(7119):1365–1368.

5. Goy E, Ganzini L. End-of-life care in geriatric psychiatry. *Clin Geriatr Med*. Nov 2003;19(4): vii-viii, 841–856.

6. Common psychiatric disorders. In: Holland JC GD, Hughes MK, eds. *Quick Reference for Oncology Clinicians: The Psychological Dimensions of Cancer Symptom Management*: Charlottesville, VA: American Psychosocial Oncology Society Institute for Research and Education; 2006.

7. Roth AJ, Komblith AB, Batel-Copel L, et al. Rapid screening for psychologic distress in men with prostate carcinoma: a pilot study. *Cancer*. 1998;82(10):1904–1908.

8. Jacobsen PB, Donovan KA, Trask PC, et al. Screening for psychologic distress in ambulatory cancer patients. *Cancer*. 2005;103(7):1494–1502.

9. Levin T, Y A. Anxiety disorders. In: Holland JBW, Jacobsen PB, Lederberg M, Loscalzo M, McCorkle R, eds. *Psycho-Oncology*. 2nd ed. New York, NY: Oxford University Press; 2010:324–330.

10. Jacobsen PB, Bovbjerg DH, Redd WH. Anticipatory anxiety in women receiving chemotherapy for breast cancer. *Health psychology: official journal of the Division of Health Psychology, American Psychological Association*. Nov 1993;12(6):469–475.

11. Portenoy RK, Thaler HT, Kornblith AB, et al. The Memorial Symptom Assessment Scale: an instrument for the evaluation of symptom prevalence, characteristics and distress. *Europe J Cancer*. 1994;30A(9):1326–1336.

12. Chang VT, Hwang SS, Feuerman M. Validation of the Edmonton Symptom Assessment Scale. *Cancer*. May 1 2000;88(9):2164–2171.

13. Zigmond AS, Snaith RP. The hospital anxiety and depression scale. *Acta psychiatrica Scandinavica*. June 1983;67(6):361–370.

14. Derogatis LR, Melisaratos N. The Brief Symptom Inventory: an introductory report. *Psychologic Med*. Aug 1983;13(3):595–605.

15. Speilberger CD. *Manual for the State-Trait Anxiety Inventory (Form Y)*. Palo Alto, CA: Consulting Psychologists Press; 1983.

16. Spitzer RL, Kroenke K, Williams JB, Lowe B. A brief measure for assessing generalized anxiety disorder: the GAD-7. *Arch Intern Med*. May 22 2006;166 (10):1092–1097.

17. *Diagnostic and Statistical Manual of Mental Disorders*. 5th ed. Arlington, VA: American Psychiatric Association; 2013.

18. Roth AJ, Modi R. Psychiatric issues in older cancer patients. *Crit Revs in Oncol/Hematol.* 2003;48:185–197.

19. Passik SD, Roth AJ. Anxiety symptoms and panic attacks preceding pancreatic cancer diagnosis. *Psycho-oncol.* May-Jun 1999;8(3):268–272.

20. Miller K, Massie MJ. Depressive disorders. In: Holland J, Breitbart W, Jacobsen PB, Lederberg M, Loscalzo M, McCorkle R, eds. *Psycho-Oncology.* 2nd ed. New York, NY: Oxford University Press; 2010:311–318.

21. Katon W, Lin E, Kroenke K. The association of depression and anxiety with medical symptom burden in patients with chronic medical illness. *Gen Hosp Psychiat.* 2007;147–155.

22. Rao A, Cohen HJ. Symptom management in the elderly cancer patient: fatigue, pain, and pepression. *J Natl Cancer Inst.* 2004;32:150–157.

23. NCCN. Distress management. *The Complete Library of NCCN Clinical Practice Guidelines in Oncology.* Jenkintown, PA: National Comprehensive Cancer Network; 2008.

Chapter 8

Substance-Use Disorders in Older Adults with Chronic Cancer Pain

Adam Rzetelny, Matthew Ruehle, Nicholas Miller,
Kenneth L. Kirsh, and Steven D. Passik

Overview

Over the last decade or two, the public-health crisis of chronic pain in our aging society has led to a dramatic increase in the prescribing of opioids and other controlled substances. A parallel set of public-health crises has arisen that include the problems of prescription-drug abuse, diversion of drugs, overdose, and death. Up to 85 percent of substance-use disorders (SUDs), are manifest by the age of 35,[1] whereas cancer has increasingly become a disease of those 50 and older. Although an older person with pain from cancer is highly unlikely to develop addiction de novo in this context,[2] increasing percentages of older Americans have a history of drug use in the remote or recent past. There is greater opportunity for those who come to the disease with a history of SUD to lose control, overuse, or even have the problem of addiction fully rekindled.[3] Finally, of additional concern for those prescribing controlled substances and treating pain (or anxiety and other symptoms) in older people, their medications are increasingly sought after by younger drug abusers in their family or environment (everyone from their grandchildren to those helping to care for them).

Many of the painful illnesses affecting older people, including cancer, have been transformed into chronic diseases. Thus opioid exposure for an older person could go on for years. If that older person comes to their cancer illness with a history of SUD, there is ample time (and stress) for old problems to be rekindled or ongoing problems exacerbated. If there are people in their social context who would borrow, share, or steal their medications, these patients can become targets of diversion. Thus, the management of cancer pain, including pain in older adults, must begin with an appreciation for these risks on the part of the clinician and proceed following risk stratification, and in the context of a risk management paradigm. Though alcohol remains one of the most abused and problematic drugs in older adults, as in any age group, the focus of this chapter is the use of illicit drugs and the misuse, abuse, and potential for diversion of prescription medications among older adults with cancer.

The terms *substance-use disorder* (SUD) and addiction are used interchangeably but are not necessarily identical, and continue to cause confusion among many health-care professionals and the patients they treat. Although addiction is the more traditional and familiar term, SUD is the more recent and preferred term used in the fifth edition of the *Diagnostic and Statistical Manual*.[4]

Scope of the Problem and Trends

The number of illicit drug users aged 50 years or older is expected to approximately double from 2000 to 2020 because of an anticipated 52 percent increase in this segment of the population and the attendant shift in attitudes and historical experiences with substance use in this cohort.[5] Among adults aged 50 or older, nearly 5 million, or a little more than 5 percent of that age group, report using illicit drugs in the past year.[6] Marijuana is the most abused drug in the U.S., but among adults aged 60 or older, the abuse of prescription drugs is equally common. As people age, the social incentive to smoke marijuana decreases, whereas the attempt to use it medicinally increases. In the oncology setting, this might include an attempt to self-medicate nausea, anorexia, pain, anxiety, or combinations of these common symptoms. Emergency room visits related to pharmaceutical abuse more than doubled from 2004 to 2008 among adults aged 50 or older, and a fifth of these were among adults aged 70 or older.[7] Prescription-opioids were the most common, followed by benzodiazepines. Alcohol is the only substance of abuse being treated that decreased from 87.6 to 58.0 percent, whereas the addition of other drugs to alcohol increased from 12.4 to 42.0 percent. Treatment admissions involving heroin more than doubled, from 7.2 to 16.0 percent, and those reporting multiple drugs of abuse nearly tripled.[8] Although family and friends remain the most frequent sources of diverted prescription medications,[9] health-care professionals are much more likely to represent an inadvertant source of diversion among older adults in substance-treatment settings (>60%) relative to younger adults (~30%).[1]

There is a paucity of information on older patients and the risk of comorbid pain and SUDs. Inadequate pain management can lead to alternative methods for relieving pain such as taking nonprescribed medications.[10,11] Though severe chronic pain is common in adults who enter treatment for prescription opioid abuse, it is exponentially more prevalent in adults older than 45 years (70%) relative to adults aged 18–24 (45%).[1]

Patterns of Use by the Elderly
Early-onset users:
- More prevalent.
- Have a long history of substance abuse.
- Continue to abuse illicit drugs even as they age.[12]

Late-onset users, (less than 10%)
- Develop the habit when older.
- High rates of painful medical conditions.
- Self-medication.
- Depression.
- Dementia.
- Cognitive impairment.
- Social isolation.
- Poor support systems.[13]

Data obtained
Risk Factors for Substance Use Disorders
- Female gender.
- Social isolation.
- History of substance abuse.
- History of mental illness.
- Medical exposure to prescription drugs with abuse potential.
- "Young" elder (age 50–60).
- Unmarried male.
- Low income status.
- Current methadone maintenance.
- Substance abuse among close contacts.
- Involvement in crime, especially drug crime.[14,15,16,17,18]

Additional Risks for SUD in the Older Cancer Patient
- Potential drug interactions
- Polypharmacy is likely warranted in the older person with cancer.
- Greater drug sensitivity in older adults,[17] especially those undergoing chemotherapies and other cancer treatments.

Opioids and benzodiazepines are commonly prescribed in the elderly and can cause respiratory depression or increase the risk of falls. These risks can be multiplied in the presence of unmonitored dose escalations, heroin, benzodiazepine, or alcohol abuse. Cocaine or other stimulant abuse can exacerbate the risk of dysrhythmias such as QT prolongation, especially in patients already being treated for cardiac conditions.

Awareness of potentially reduced cytochrome P450 metabolic enzyme activity in the elderly and, thus, increased risk for drug-drug interactions is imperative. Inhibitory medications include common antidepressants such as fluoxetine and paroxetine, antiarrhythmics such as quinidine, proton-pump inhibitors, antibiotics such as clarithromycin, and antifungals such as ketoconazole (for a list of P450 substrates, inhibitors, and inducers, go to http://medicine.iupui.edu/clinpharm/ddis/main-table/; for an FDA list of medication labels that include P450 cautions, warnings, or dosage adjustments, go to http://www.fda.gov/Drugs/ScienceResearch/ResearchAreas/Pharmacogenetics/ucm083378.htm). Genetic abnormalities, or polymorphisms, can seriously complicate the already elevated risk of drug interactions in elderly pain populations.

Principles and Practices of Substance Abuse Care of the Elderly Cancer Patient

• Be careful not to be overly suspicious of patients.
• Neither assume they are immune from aberrant behaviors.
• Older patient may suffer pain and despair because of fear of SUD.
• Oncology professionals need to educate and dispel fear.
• Assess and protect those who need to have controlled substances.
• Clarify what is and is not an SUD.
  • SUDs are not merely physiological dependence: expected biological adaptation to continuous exposure.
  • The hallmarks of dependence are tolerance and withdrawal.
  • Tolerance is the expected gradual dose increases sometimes needed to maintain the desired therapeutic effect
  • Withdrawal is a set of adverse symptoms experienced upon abrupt or rapid discontinuation.

Symptoms of withdrawal

• flu-like syndrome.
• Nervousness.
• Excessive yawning and goose bumps.

Gradual discontinuation of medications is recommended. Cancer patients might need to decrease or taper opioids, for example, after an acutely painful period or after exacerbation of their cancer is treated and the pain associated with it diminishes (such as the treatment of a painful bone metastasis with radiation therapy). Thus, dependence is not a sign that the pain patient is becoming addicted.

SUDs, likewise, are not defined merely by physiologic tolerance, which also is a normal development that follows upon continuous exposure (though the time period varies from days to weeks from person to person).

Tolerance refers to the need to increase the drug to maintain the desired effect, such as pain relief. Tolerance is highly variable in people with pain, and requests for higher doses need to be evaluated carefully. The need for some adjustment in dose over time is not a sign that the patient is becoming addicted. Because tolerance develops not only to the pain-relieving aspects of the drugs, but also to side effects like sedation and the slowing down of one's breathing, the dose of opioids can be continually raised for patients suffering with progressive and debilitating conditions over time. Misconceptions of tolerance often lead people with cancer to suffer because they are afraid that they need to save their pain medicines for when they really need them. SUDs, or addiction, is often indicated by craving a substance that is used in an unrestrained, often compulsive manner, despite harm.

Assessment

Assessment Tools

10 steps of Universal Precautions in Older Patients with opioid therapy[19,20]

- Reasonable attempts to make a diagnosis with an appropriate differential.
- Comprehensive patient assessment including risk of addictive disorders.
- Informed consent.
- Treatment agreement.
- Pre- and postintervention assessment of pain level and function.
- Appropriate trial of opioid therapy ± "adjunctive" medications.
- Reassessment of pain score and level of function.
- Regular assessment of the four A's of pain medicine (Analgesia; Activities of daily living; Adverse effects; and Aberrant drug-related behaviors).
- Periodic review of pain diagnosis and comorbid conditions and addictive disorders.
- Documentation.

Prescribers should utilize brief screening tools when choosing candidates for opioid therapies. This can be helpful for identifying patients that they can treat alone, those whom they can treat with help, and those whom they must refer to other specialists. Most validated instruments for SUDs in older adults are focused on alcohol, and some of these may be useful, though to a limited degree, for assessing other substances of abuse. Still, research related to the Brief Intervention and Treatment for Elders (BRITE) (a version of Screening, Brief Intervention, and Referral to Treatment (SBIRT) that is more geared toward the elderly) shows that assessment options for the aged may be on the rise and provide unique utility.[21] At a minimum, a tool such as the CAGE, adapted for potential illicit or prescription substance abuse, may be appropriate as a screening tool, as it is particularly brief and entirely verbal, conducted during an interview or in the course of impromptu conversation.

An objective assessment tool widely utilized in settings where controlled substances are prescribed, and an important component of universal precautions is urine or oral-fluid testing (henceforth referred to as urine drug testing; UDT). UDT is initially an assessment tool but can become part of ongoing monitoring during the management phase.

Interviews

The interview process should include risk factors such as age at first use of all substances including tobacco, and not just opioids. Obtaining a detailed history in a nonjudgmental empathic and truthful manner about duration, frequency, and desired effect of drug use is vital.[22,23]

In anticipating defensiveness on the part of the patient, it can be helpful for clinicians to mention that patients often misrepresent their drug use for logical reasons, such as stigmatization, mistrust of the interviewer, or concerns regarding fears of under treatment. It is also wise for clinicians to explain that in an effort to keep the patient as comfortable as possible, by preventing withdrawal states and prescribing sufficient medication for pain and symptom control, an accurate account of drug use is necessary.

This approach begins with broad and general inquiries regarding the role of drugs in the patient's life, such as caffeine and nicotine, and gradually proceeds to more specific questions regarding illicit drugs. This interview style can also assist in discerning any coexisting psychiatric disorders, which can significantly contribute to aberrant drug-taking behavior. Once identified, treatment of comorbid psychiatric disorders can greatly enhance management strategies and decrease the risk of relapse.

Management/Treatment/Prevention

Because abuse of illicit and prescription drugs among older adults is on the rise—the so-called "hidden" or "silent" epidemic—enhanced efforts aimed at identifying and treating nonalcohol SUDs are needed.[17] It is incumbent upon primary health-care and other medical professionals, including oncologists, to embrace their increasing role as the "front line" in addressing the problem. This involves greater awareness of prevalence, risks, and patterns that can lead to proactive identification, and being ready with age-appropriate management and treatment responses, including a risk-stratified approach to identifying which individuals can be managed in the primary health-care setting, co-managed, or referred to specialty treatment.

There is a dearth of information on the challenges of treatment for elderly SUDs. Pope.[24] has noted that family participation remains significant even into older adulthood.

When beginning medication-assisted substance-abuse treatment with the elderly, the clinician must take into consideration all medical comorbidities, start medications at low doses and utilize a slow titration to effect.

Risk Stratified Management and Treatment

Older adults with late onset SUDs may respond adequately to simple education and monitoring strategies, whereas the early-onset type will likely require a more comprehensive approach.[12] Additionally, there may be greater fear and reluctance to admit drug problems or accept help among older adults. In all cases, once an older patient has been appropriately assessed and his or her degree of risk ascertained, management begins with frank and nonjudgmental communication with the patient about the potential risks and benefits of various treatments, including the risks of misuse, abuse, and diversion associated with controlled substances.

The cognitive status of the older cancer patient must be taken into account when estimating his or her ability to understand and remember education about the risks and benefits of treatment, what is expected of them as a patient for self-report of medication adherence, changes in disease state, or functioning. In some cases, inclusion of family members involved in the patient's treatment should be considered.

Summary and Conclusion

Pain management in older cancer patients must begin with an appreciation for the risks of SUDs and diversion in these populations that have grown in recent years. Although there is a lack of data pertaining to the components of a risk-management paradigm, in general, and specifically to how it applies to older cancer patients with pain, a clinician can and should apply techniques and tools that have shown promise in the management of the younger person with pain. Our duty to treat pain safely and effectively for the patient, and to do so in a way that also protects the community against diversion, mandates that elements of this approach be adopted. In the end, when done well, this approach may lead to satisfying outcomes even in some highly challenging clinical situations.

References

1. Cicero TJ., Surratt HL, Kurtz S, Ellis, MS, Inciardi, JA. Patterns of prescription opioid abuse and co-morbidity in an aging treatment population. *J Subst Abuse Treat.*2012;42(1):87–94.

2. Minozzi S, Amato L, Davoli M. Development of dependence following treatment with opioid analgesics for pain relief: a systematic review. *Addiction.* 2013 Apr;108(4):688–698.

3. Modesto-Lowe V, Girard L, Chaplin M. Cancer pain in the opioid-addicted patient: can we treat it right? *J Opioid Manag.* 2012;8(3):167–175.

4. American Psychiatric Association. *Diagnostic and Statistical Manual of Mental Disorders.* 5th ed.: DSM-5, Washington DC: Author; 2013.

5. Colliver JD, Compton WM, Gfroerer J, Condon T. Projecting drug use among aging baby boomers in 2020. *Ann Epidemiol,* 2006;16:257–265.

6. SAMHSA. (2011). Substance Abuse and Mental Health Services Administration. *National Survey on Drug Use and Health: Illicit drug use among older adults.* Available at: http://www.samhsa.gov/data/2k11/WEB_SR_013/WEB_SR_013.htm

7. SAMHSA. Drug Abuse Warning Network (DAWN). *Emergency Department Visits Involving Illicit Drug Use by Older Adults: 2008.* Rockville, MD:Author; 2010.

8. SAMHSA. Substance Abuse and Mental Health Services Administration. *Treatment Episode Data Set (TEDS). Changing substance abuse patterns among older admissions: 1992 and 2008.* Rockville, MD: Author; 2010.

9. SAMHSA. Substance Abuse and Mental Health Services Administration. *Results from the 2012 National Survey on Drug Use and Health: Summary of National Findings.* Rockville, MD: Author; 2013.

10. Manchikanti L, Damron KS, McManus CD, Barnhill RC. Patterns of illicit drug use and opioid abuse in patients with chronic pain at initial evaluation: A prospective, observational study. *Pain Phys.* 2004;7:431–437.

11. Morasco B, Dobscha S. Prescription medication misuse in substance use disorder in VA primary care patients with chronic pain. *Gen Hosp Psychiat.* 2008;30:93–99.

12. Roe B, Beynon C, Pickering L, Duffy P (2010). Experience of drug use and ageing: health, quality of life, relationships and service implications. *J Adv Nurs.* 2010; 66(9):1968–1979.

13. Taylor MH, Grossberg GT (2012). The growing problem of illicit substance abuse in the elderly: A review. *Prim Care Companion CNS Disord.* 2012;14(4):pii.

14. Arndt S, Turvey CL, Flaum M. (2002). Older offenders, substance abuse, and treatment. *Am J Geriatr Psychiat.* 2002;10(6):733–739.

15. Simoni-Wastila L, Yang HK. Psychoactive drug abuse in older adults. *Am J Geriatr Pharmacother.* 2006;4(4):380–394.

16. Briggs WP, Magnus VA, Lassiter P, Patterson A, Smith L. (2011). Substance use, misuse, and abuse among older adults: Implications for clinical mental health counselors. *J Ment Health Couns.* 2011 33(2):112–127.

17. Wu L, Blazer DG. Illicit and nonmedical drug use among older adults: A review. *J Aging Health.* 2011; 23(3):481–504.

18. Rosen D, Hunsaker A, Albert SM, Cornelius JR, Reynolds CF. Characteristics and consequences of heroin use among older adults in the United States: a review of literature, treatment implications, and recommendations for further research. *Addict Behav.* 2011;36(4):279–285.

19. Gourlay DL, Heit HA. Universal precautions in pain medicine: a rational approach to the treatment of chronic pain. *Pain Med.* 2005;6:107.

20. Gourlay D, Heit H. Universal precautions: a matter of mutual trust and responsibility. *Pain Med.* 2006;7(2):210–212.

21. Schonfeld L, King-Kallimanis BL, Duchene DM, Etheridge RL, Herrera JR, Barry K L, Lynn N. Screening and brief intervention for substance misuse among older adults: The Florida BRITE project. *American Journal of Public Health.* 2010;100(1):108–114.

22. Passik SD, Portenoy RK. Substance abuse disorders. In: Holland JC. *Psycho-Oncology.* New York, NY: Oxford University Press; 1998: 576–586.

23. Savage SR, Kirsh KL, Passik SD. Challenges in using opioids to treat pain in persons with substance use disorders. *Addiction Science & Clinical Practice.* 2008;4(2):4–25. Retrieved from http://www.drugabuse.gov/PDF/ascp/vol4no2/Challenges.pdf

24. Pope RC, Wallhagen M, Davis H. The social determinants of substance abuse in African American baby boomers: effects of family, media images, and environment. *J Transcult Nurs,* 2010;21(3):246–256.

Chapter 9

Personality Disorders in Older Cancer Patients

Kenneth L. Kirsh, Steven D. Passik, and Andrew J. Roth

Introduction

Personality disorders are life long ways of thinking and feeling about oneself and others that affects how an individual functions in many aspects of life. These enduring traits can have adverse or maladaptive consequences in interpersonal relationships, often worsening during health crisis like cancer and leading to problematic or confrontation encounters with health-care givers. The prevalence of personality disorders among older people in the community has been estimated to be about 10 percent.[1] Personality disorders or subsyndromal personality psychopathology can affect the overall functioning and quality of life of elders living either independently or in institutional settings.[2]

The fifth edition of the *Diagnostic and Statistical Manual of Mental Disorders*[3] has re-organized clinical assessment of the different aspects and impact of all mental, personality, and other medical disorders from a multi-axial system into a single axis classification. Personality disorders in older people are often comorbid with anxiety and depression disorders,[4] making diagnosis that much more complicated.

It has been helpful to think about personality disorders as placed into 3 clusters: the odd, paranoid or eccentric; the avoidant, dependent, and anxious; and the impulsive/self-centered or flamboyant. It is felt that those in the first two clusters may become less functional and experience more difficulty over time as they age, whereas those in the last cluster, except for borderlines, having better lives as they age.[5]

Older cancer patients with personality disorders who face the anxiety and discomfort associated with medical treatment can have difficulties with medical caregivers, distort reality for emotional protection, or exhibit outright aggression and self-destructiveness.[6]

An increase in obsessive–compulsive traits is common among older people and may reflect not so much a change in intrinsic personality as an adaptation of the person to failing powers or altered relationships and environments.[7] See Box 9.1, Tables 9.1 and 9.2, and Figure 9.1.

Box 9.1 Key Attributes of Personality Disorder

- A consistent pattern of behaviors that deviates markedly from the expectations of the individual's culture.
- Stable over time.
- Pervasive and inflexible.
- Has onset in adolescence or early adulthood.
- Thought to be poor coping or defense mechanisms used to buffer residual high stress that has not been overcome.
- Leads to distrust or impairment.

Table 9.1 Types of Personality Disorders and Their Key Components

Paranoid	• Suspicious of others • Perceives attacks by others quickly • Categorizes people as an enemy or friend • Rarely confides in others • Unforgiving
Schizoid	• Flat affect • Tends to be solitary in nature • Indifferent to criticism and praise • Marked absence of close friends or relationships
Schizotypal	• Has magical thinking or odd beliefs • Exhibits anxiety in social situations • Paranoid ideation • Experiences unusual perceptions
Antisocial	• Lacks conformity to laws • Ignores obligations • Impulsive • Irritable and aggressive
Borderline	• Fears of abandonment • Suicidal behavior • Mood instability • Chronic feelings of emptiness
Histrionic	• Easily influenced • Rapidly shifting emotions • Theatrical emotions • Provocative or sexual behavior
Narcissistic	• Belief in being "special" • Lacks empathy • Arrogant • Sense of entitlement

(continued)

Table 9.1 (Continued)

Avoidant	• Self view as inferior • Inhibited in new relationships • Tries to avoid embarrassment • Fear of rejection in social situations
Dependent	• Fears of being left alone • Lack of self-confidence • Requires reassurance when making decisions • Unlikely to express disagreement for fear of rejection
Obsessive-Compulsive	• Preoccupied with details • Tendency for perfectionism • Inflexible and stubborn • Unable to discard worthless objects
Personality Disorder NOS	• Reserved for disorders that do not fit any of the other categories • Can also describe people who exhibit features of several personality disorders without meeting full criteria for any one disorder

Adapted from Eysenck H. The definition of personality disorders and the criteria appropriate for their descriptions. *J Pers Disord*. 1987;1:211–219; Pinkofsky HB. Mnemonics for *DSM-IV* personality disorders. Psychiatric Services (Washington, DC). Sep 1997;48(9):1197–1198.

Table 9.2 Personality Disorder Screening and Evaluation

Taking a psychological history	• Be straightforward in assessing a taboo subject. • Those with past history of psychological distress or personality disorders are more likely to suffer from both in the future. • Personality disorders are difficult to diagnose. • Significant comorbidity exists among personality disorders. • Comorbidity leads to difficulty in identifying a primary personality diagnosis. • Axis I disorders will complicate the identification of personality disorders.[10,11]
The physician's perspective	• The clinician with the personality-disordered patient does not need to make the diagnosis to be successful, but he or she must respond to the behavior. • Avoid stereotyping patients. • Be aware of your own feelings towards your patients, especially those who cause you to have emotional reactions.
Make a referral to a Mental Health Provider: social worker, psychologist, or psychiatrist, depending on what is available in your community/organization.*	• Cancer patients utilize mental health professionals more often than the general public (7.2% versus 5.7%).[12] • When a patient is challenging the resources of the physician and staff, it is a wise decision to enroll the aid of a mental health provider.

* It is always useful to establish a relationship in your practice with mental health providers. They should have an understanding and respect for the challenges of dealing with cancer patients who also have a comorbid personality disorder. Frequent feedback and discussion of the patient's status is helpful to all involved.

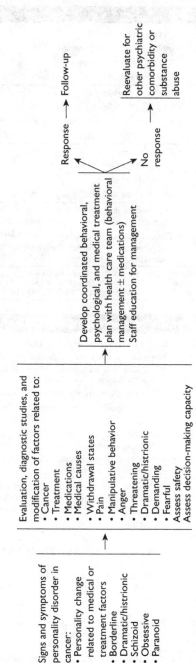

Figure 9.1 NCCN Distress Management Guidelines DIS-17–Personality Disorder. Adapted from Personality Disorder (DIS-17). Reproduced with permission from the NCCN 1.2005 Distress Management, *The Complete Library of NCCN Clinical Practice Guidelines in Oncology* [CD-Rom]. May 2005.

Interventions

Treatments for personality disorders are shown in Table 9.3.

Brief Intervention—The FRAMES Technique

Physicians can often feel unnerved by dealing with difficult patients who have personality disorders. They may begin to avoid interactions with the patients and feel that they always end in confrontations. The following FRAMES (Feedback, Responsibility, Advice, Menu, Empathy) technique is a handy way to structure contacts with these patients while delivering needed information in a structured way. See Table 9.4.

The Angry Patient

It is very common for patients with personality disorders to exhibit their frustrations and to take their anger out on staff and other health-care team members. The following tips are useful to prevent escalation of the patient's outbursts and escalation of staff anger and frustration. Ultimately, the goal is to help the patients to regain control and to learn to cope better with the issues that face them.

Table 9.3 Personality Disorder Treatments

Management of the psychiatric disorder	• The therapist will work on limit setting and behavior modification with patient and staff. • The physician and other health-care staff need to remember the frame of treatment and not be dragged into covering too many psychosocial issues and crises. • At times, it might be necessary to develop a signed agreement with the patient about this frame of treatment and what limits are in place with various members of the treating team.
Psychopharmacology	• Although personality disorder is best treated with psychotherapy and minimization of patient opportunity to manipulate care, there is a limited role for pharmacotherapy for specific issues. Consider the following to address features that might accompany the personality disorder: • Mood disorders (antidepressants or lithium). • Psychotic symptoms (antipsychotics). • Anxiety symptoms (anxiolytics or antipsychotics). • Possible expanded role for atypical antipsychotics.
Management of the impact of the patient's behavior on staff behavior	• Management of staff issues is critical. • Staff meetings with all those involved in the patient's care can be very helpful. • New responses to the patient's behaviors can be planned. • Maintain teamwork to manage difficult patients. • Avoiding staff splitting (i.e., do not let the patient "tell stories" about other staff members in order to create staff tension and distrust among the health-care team).

Table 9.4 The FRAMES Technique

Feedback	• Deliver information. • Make observations. • Be nonjudgmental, nonblaming. • Identify behaviors indicative of abuse and addiction; use checklists.
Responsibility	• Remind the patient that they have a role in their treatment that may be hampered by their behavior: "I am concerned that you have two problems—your cancer and possibly a problem dealing with stress." (or substance abuse/depression/anxiety . . .) • Treatment for the problem is the patient's responsibility: • "Think about what I have said." • "Observe your behaviors." • "Make a decision about your treatment."
Advice	• Offer advice from the stance of expert medical opinion instead of reward/punishment or referent authority. • Use a neutral tone: "You could take your MRI to another physician and get more drugs, but I do not advise this."
Menu	• Offer multiple treatment choices (and identify whether there are multiple problems). • Will assist with finding the best option for them. • "You may not be ready now, but I will be here for you if you change your mind at some point in the future."
Empathy	• "I know that you have been through a lot." • Patients do not consciously choose to become addicted, adopt the sick role, become depressed, etc. • Use understanding, compassion, insight.
Self-Efficacy	• Without blame, empathy becomes easier. • "I know this is very hard but I also know that you can do this." • Repeat any strengths patient has revealed by report and by your observations. • Ends intervention on a positive note. • Re-emphasize that responsibility belongs to the patient.

Box 9.2 Management of the Angry Patient

• Do not personalize.
• Listen to their perspective.
• Acknowledge their view.
• Check for accuracy, listen for feelings, listen for the underlying problem.
• Empathize.
• Reframe.

(continued)

Box 9.2 (Continued)

- Focus on different interpretations rather than "truth" (i.e., we see things differently).
- Focus on responsibility rather than blame.
- Focus on intentions and outcomes rather than accusations.
- Be clear about your decisions.
- Share your perspective—with clarity.
- Ask for feedback.
- Problem solve.
- Remember, not everyone will be happy.
- Retreat (find a colleague if necessary).
- Reevaluate.
- Re-approach.
- Make another appointment if necessary.

References

1. Abrams RC, Horowitz SV. Personality disorders after age 50: a meta-analysis. *J Pers Disord.* 1996;10:271–281.

2. Abrams RC, Bromberg C. Personality disorders in the elderly. *Psychiatr Ann.* 2007;37(2):1013–1017.

3. American Psychiatric Association. Personality Disorders Fact Sheet - DSM-5. 2014; http://www.dsm5.org/Documents/Personalitydisodersfactsheet.pdf

4. Mordekar A, Spence S. Personality disorder in older people: how common is it and what can be done? *Adv Psychiatr Treat.* 2008;14:71–77.

5. Seivewright H, Tyrer P, Johnson T. Change in personality status in neurotic disorders. *Lancet.* June 29 2002;359(9325):2253–2254.

6. Hay JL, Passik SD. The cancer patient with borderline personality disorder: suggestions for symptom-focused management in the medical setting. *Psycho-Oncol.* Mar-Apr 2000;9(2):91–100.

7. Engels GI, Duijsens IJ, Haringsma R, van Putten CM. Personality disorders in the elderly compared to four younger age groups: a cross-sectional study of community residents and mental health patients. *J Pers Disord.* Oct 2003;17(5):447–459.

8. Eysenck H. The definition of personality disorders and the criteria appropriate for their descriptions. *J Pers Disord.* 1987;1:211–219.

9. Pinkofsky HB. Mnemonics for *DSM-IV* personality disorders. *Psychiatric Services (Washington, D.).* Sep 1997;48(9):1197–1198.

10. Fishbain DA. Approaches to treatment decisions for psychiatric comorbidity in the management of the chronic pain patient. *Med Clin N Am.* May 1999;83(3):vii, 737–760.

11. Melartin TK, Rytsala HJ, Leskela US, Lestela-Mielonen PS, Sokero TP, Isometsa ET. Current comorbidity of psychiatric disorders among DSM-IV major depressive disorder patients in psychiatric care in the Vantaa Depression Study. *J Clin Psychiat.* Feb 2002;63(2):126–134.

12. Hewitt M, Rowland JH. Mental health service use among adult cancer survivors: analyses of the National Health Interview Survey. *J Clin Oncol.* Dec 1 2002;20(23):4581–4590.

Physical Symptom Management

Chapter 10

Fatigue

Daisuke Fujisawa and William F. Pirl

Introduction

Definition: Cancer-related fatigue is a distressing, persistent, subjective sense of physical, emotional, and/or cognitive tiredness or exhaustion related to cancer or cancer treatment that is not proportional to recent activity and interferes with usual functioning.[1]

Prevalence: Fatigue is experienced by 14 to 96 percent of patients undergoing cancer treatment and in 19 to 82 percent of patients posttreatment. Fatigue persists for months or even years after treatments.[2]

Impact: Fatigue is the symptom that cancer patients report most frequently and describe as the most distressing. It is associated with debilitating impact on functioning, desire for hastened death, and burden on caregivers.[3]

Specific consideration to geriatric population: There is some evidence that fatigue increases with age, but this difference is confounded by hemoglobin (Hgb) levels.[4] Little empirical evidence exists to support that cancer-related fatigue differs among populations of elderly patients and younger patients. However, elderly patients are likely to have more comorbidities and a greater number of medications, which can worsen fatigue. Most of the clinical trials that studied fatigue included but did not specifically target the geriatric population.[5]

Screening

National Comprehensive Cancer Network (NCCN) recommends screening patients for fatigue at their initial visit and then regularly with a one-item screening question:[6]

> "Since your last visit, how would you rate your worst fatigue on a scale of 0 to 10?"

Screening should be followed by education, evaluation, and general strategies to manage fatigue (see Figure 10.1). Other validated fatigue screening tools may include: Edmonton Symptom Assessment Scale (ESAS)—fatigue subscale, Brief Fatigue Inventory (BFI), Fatigue Symptom Inventory (FSI), and the Functional Assessment of Chronic Illness Therapy-Fatigue Scale (FACIT-F). See Figure 10.1.

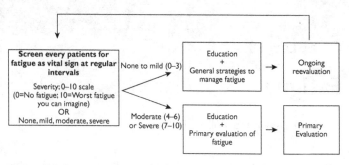

Figure 10.1 Screening.

Box 10.1 Focused History

- Disease status and treatment:
  - Rule out recurrence or progression of the cancer.
  - Relation to cancer treatments.
  - Review prescription medications/over-the-counter drugs (OTCs), and supplements.
- Review of systems (both physical and psychological).
- In-depth fatigue history:
  - Onset, pattern, duration.
  - Change over time.
  - Associated (alleviating and exacerbating) factors.
  - Interference with function.
- Social support status/availability of caregivers:
  - Impact on relationships.
  - Response to past interventions.

Primary Evaluation

Primary evaluation includes taking focused history (see Box 10.1) and assessing contributing factors (Box 10.2). Depression is one of important differential diagnoses (see Table 10.1).

Interventions

General Strategies for Management of Fatigue

If any of the previously mentioned contributing factors are identified, they should be addressed as a first step. Although some approaches to managing fatigue are relevant to all patients, others should be tailored to the patients' clinical status (on active cancer treatment/at posttreatment with no active treatment except hormonal therapy/at end of life). See Figure 10.2 and Box 10.3.

Box 10.2 Assessment of Contributing Factors

- Medications/side effects.
- Pain.
- Emotional distress:
  - Depression.
  - Anxiety.
  - Demoralization.
- Sleep disturbance (insomnia, depression, narcolepsy, obstructive sleep apnea, restless leg syndrome, akathisia).
- Anemia.
- Nutritional deficits/imbalance:
  - Weight/caloric intake changes.
  - Fluid electrolyte imbalance: sodium, potassium, calcium, magnesium.
- Decreased functional status:
  - Decreased activity level.
  - Deconditioning.
- Comorbidities:
  - Alcohol/substance abuse.
  - Cardiac dysfunction.
  - Endocrine dysfunction (e.g., hot flashes, hypothyroidism, hypogonadism, adrenal insufficiency).
    - These can be caused by surgery, radiation therapy/chemotherapy/hormonal therapy:
  - Gastrointestinal dysfunction.
  - Hepatic dysfunction.
  - Infection.
  - Neurologic dysfunction (including hypoactive delirium).
  - Pulmonary dysfunction.
  - Renal dysfunction.

Table 10.1 Distinguishing Fatigue from Depression

Fatigue	Patients usually are able to derive some pleasure from activities that they normally find enjoyable and have goals to accomplish were their fatigue to subside.
	Late afternoon is the most difficult time of the day.
Depression	Patients are unable to experience pleasure from experiences that they usually enjoy.
	Morning is the most difficult time of the day and have few goals should their fatigue subside.
	Past history and/or family history of major depression may increase the likelihood of developing an episode of depression.

Note: Fatigue and depression may be concurrent. In cases of uncertainty, an empiric trial of antidepressant therapy (i.e., and energizing antidepressant such as bupropion) may be considered in order not to let a possible case of depression go untreated. Depressive syndromes can be even more difficult to recognize in the elderly than in younger patients.

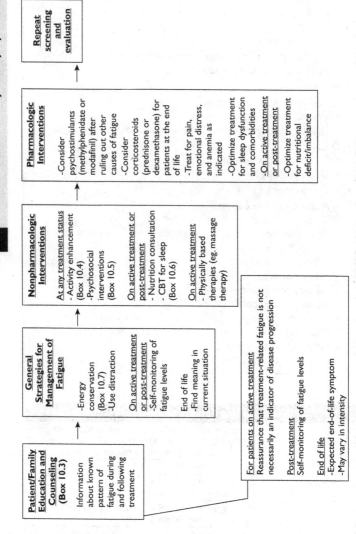

Patient/Family Education and Counseling (Box 10.3)

Information about known pattern of fatigue during and following treatment

General Strategies for Management of Fatigue

-Energy conservation (Box 10.7)
-Use distraction

On active treatment or post-treatment
-Self-monitoring of fatigue levels

End of life
-Find meaning in current situation

Nonpharmacologic Interventions

At any treatment status
- Activity enhancement (Box 10.4)
-Psychosocial interventions (Box 10.5)

On active treatment or post-treatment
- Nutrition consultation
- CBT for sleep (Box 10.6)

On active treatment
- Physically based therapies (eg. massage therapy)

Pharmacologic Interventions

-Consider psychostimulants (methylphenidate or modafinil) after ruling out other causes of fatigue
-Consider corticosteroids (prednisone or dexamethasone) for patients at the end of life
-Treat for pain, emotional distress, and anemia as indicated
-Optimize treatment for sleep dysfunction and comorbidities
-On active treatment or post-treatment
-Optimize treatment for nutritional deficit/imbalance

Repeat screening and evaluation

For patients on active treatment
Reassurance that treatment-related fatigue is not necessarily an indicator of disease progression

Post-treatment
Self-monitoring of fatigue levels

End of life
-Expected end-of-life symptom
-May vary in intensity

Figure 10.2 Interventions.

Box 10.3 Patient and Family Education and Counseling

- All cancer patients should be provided with education about fatigue and its natural history.
- For patients on active treatment:
  - Education is essential for patients initiating potentially fatigue-inducing treatments before the onset of fatigue.
  - Reassure that treatment-related fatigue is not necessarily an indicator of disease progression.
  - Baseline and ongoing daily self-monitoring of fatigue levels in a treatment log or diary may be helpful to identify patterns and triggers.
- For patients at posttreatment phase:
  - Inform patients that a significant subset of patients continue to experience distressing levels of fatigue; however, most patients experience a gradual decrease in fatigue and return of energy to normal levels.
  - Encourage regular self-monitoring of fatigue levels to document the decrease of fatigue.
- For patients at end-of-life period:
  - Patients and families need to be apprised of fatigue as an expected end-of-life symptom, so that they can begin planning for it.
  - Active commitment by the health-care team to palliative care is critical when aggressive cancer therapy is given to those with a low likelihood of long-term survival.

Nonpharmacologic Interventions

Activity enhancement (Box 10.4) and psychosocial interventions (Box 10.5) are recommended for patients at any treatment status. Meta-analytical reviews have shown that physical exercise reduces fatigue during and after cancer therapy.[7] Nutrition consultation (adequate hydration and electrolyte balance, and consult for nutritionist) and cognitive behavioral therapy for sleep (Box 10.6) are recommended as indicated for patients in active treatment or posttreatment. There is some evidence supporting the efficacy of physically based therapies (massage therapy, acupuncture) for patients in active treatment. There is no robust evidence for nonpharmacologic interventions at the end of life; however, clinicians are encouraged to consider matching the patient with activity enhancement or psychosocial intervention as indicated. See Boxes 10.4–10.6.

Many patients benefit from energy conservation and use of distraction and engagement. Energy conservation is a deliberately planned management of one's personal resources to prevent energy depletion. (See Box 10.7.) Although energy conservation may be helpful, it is important to remain as physically active as possible given the strong data on exercise. Descriptive studies have also suggested that activities designed to distract

Box 10.4 Activity Enhancement (Physical Exercise)

- Maintain optimal level of activity.
- Consider starting and maintain an exercise program, as appropriate per health-care provider, of both endurance exercises (walking, jogging, or swimming) and resistance exercises (light weights).
  - E.g., Moderately intense exercise (55–75% of heart rate), aerobic exercise ranging from 10 to 90 minutes in duration 3 to 7 days per week.
- Exercise program should be individualized based on the patient's physical and clinical backgrounds, starting at a low level of intensity and duration, progressing slowly and being modified as the patient's condition changes.
- Specific issues that should trigger a referral for rehabilitation specialist include:
  - Patients with comorbidities (e.g., cardiovascular disease or COPD).
  - Recent major surgery.
  - Specific functional or anatomical deficits (e.g., decreased range of motion due to neck dissection for head and neck cancer).
  - Substantial deconditioning.
- Caution in patients with any of the following:
  - Bone metastases.
  - Thrombocytopenia.
  - Anemia.
  - Fever or active infection.
  - Limitations secondary to metastasis or other illnesses.
  - Late effects of treatment (e.g., cardiomyopathy at posttreatment).
  - Assessment of safety issues (e.g., risk of falls, stability).

Box 10.5 Psychosocial Interventions

- Cognitive behavioral therapy (CBT)/Behavioral therapy (BT):
  - The CBT focuses on each participant's unique pattern of the following six possible factors that might serve to perpetuate their postcancer treatment fatigue:
    - Insufficient coping with the experience of cancer.
    - Fear of disease recurrence.
    - Dysfunctional cognitions regarding fatigue.
    - Dysregulation of sleep.
    - Dysregulation of activity.
    - Low social support/negative social interactions.
  - CBT includes cognitive therapy, relaxation techniques, counseling, social support, hypnosis, and biofeedback:
- Psycho-educational therapies/educational therapies.
- Supportive expressive therapies (especially for end-of-life patients).
- These interventions can be combined with complimentary therapies
  - e.g., relaxation [breathing control, progressive muscle relaxation, guided imagery techniques], massage therapy, yoga, mindfulness stress reduction).

Box 10.6 CBT for Sleep

- Stimulus control: going to bed only when sleepy; going to bed at approximately same time each night; getting out of bed after 20 minutes if unable to fall asleep; and maintaining a regular rising time each day.
- Sleep restriction: avoiding long or late afternoon naps and limiting total time in bed.
- Sleep hygiene: e.g., Avoiding caffeine after noon and establishing an environment that is conducive to sleep (e.g., dark, quiet, and comfortable) or evening alcohol, which may induce sleep but may lead to middle-of-the-night insomnia.

Box 10.7 Energy Conservation

- Set priorities and realistic expectations.
- Pace.
- Delegate.
- Schedule activities at times of peak energy.
- Use labor-saving devices:
  - For example, "reachers" for grasping items beyond arm's length, rolling carts for transporting items, escalators and elevators, electrical appliances for performing common household tasks.
  - For end-of-life patients, consider wheelchairs, walkers, and commodes.
- Postpone (or eliminate) nonessential activities, and conserve energy for valued activities.
- Limit naps to <1 hour to not interfere with nighttime sleep quality.
  - Patients at end of life should be allowed to take a day-time nap as long as it does not disturb night-time sleep.
- Structured daily routine.
- Attend one activity at a time.

(e.g., games, music, reading, socializing) are helpful for some patients in decreasing fatigue. For patients at the end of life, emphasis may be placed on finding meaning in their current situation, such as having meaningful interactions with their significant others and on promoting dignity of the patient.

Pharmacologic Interventions

Treatment of Anemia

A Cochrane review concluded that erythropoiesis-stimulating agents (ESAs) significantly reduce fatigue for anemic patients receiving chemotherapy[8]; however, the review conducted by the Food and Drug

Administration (FDA)[9] showed that ESAs shortened overall survival and/ or increased the risk of tumor progression or recurrence in patients with breast; non-small cell lung, head, and neck; lymphoid; and cervical cancers. ESAs also increase the risk of serious cardiovascular and thromboembolic events when they are administered to patients with higher hemoglobin levels (Hgb > 13.5–14 g/dL).

In accordance with the FDA-approved uses, ESAs should be restricted to the treatment of anemia (Hgb < 10 g/dL) due to concomitant palliative myelosuppressive chemotherapy and should be discontinued upon completion of a course of chemotherapy. The lowest possible dose should be used, with the goal of avoiding red blood cell transfusions. The FDA-approved guidelines state that ESAs are not indicated for patients receiving curative myelosuppressive chemotherapy. However, the 2010 ASCO/ASH recommendations state that clinical judgment, goals of therapy, and patient preference should guide ESA use in the curative and palliative settings.[10] The FDA mandates a risk management program to inform health-care providers and their patients about the risk of ESAs. ESAs should be discontinued if there is no response after 6 to 8 weeks (Hgb increase <1–2 g/dL) or no decrease in transfusion requirements.

Psychostimulants

Although there are anecdotal experiences on efficacies, RCTs of psychostimulants, including methylphenidate and modafinil, failed to demonstrate significant difference against placebo; however a subset analyses found benefits in patients with severe fatigue and/or advanced disease. Dexamphetamine showed short-term (day 2) improvement but no long-term (day 8) benefit.[11] The National Comprehensive Cancer Network (NCCN) guideline recommends consideration of methylphenidate or modafinil when other causes of fatigue have been excluded. Common side effects of psychostimulants are anorexia, insomnia, euphoria, headache, nausea, anxiety, and mood lability. High doses and long-term use may induce nightmares, paranoia, and possible cardiovascular complications (e.g., hypertension and tachycardia). Cardiovascular complications are thought to be less with modafinil and armodafinil (see Table 10.2). Methylphenidate and dexamphetamine may lower the seizure threshold. See Table 10.2.

Corticosteroids and Other Drugs

Corticosteroids (predonisone and dexamethasone) may be effective for short-term relief of fatigue. However, given the toxicity associated with long-term use, steroids are usually limited to the terminally ill or if the patient has concomitant anorexia and/or pain related to brain or bone metastases. A systematic review revealed no benefit of progestational steroids (e.g., megestrol).[8]

Selective serotonin reuptake inhibitor paroxetine showed no beneficial effect in treating fatigue. Bupropion may have benefit and needs to be examined in randomized controlled studies.[12] Donepezil showed no significant difference over placebo.[8] Treatment for nutritional deficit or

Table 10.2 Psychostimulants for Adult Cancer Patients

Drug	Dosage	Comments/Primary Side Effects
Dextroamphetamine (Dexedrine)	2.5 mg/d (start) 5–30 mg/d in 2 to 3 divided doses	Schedule II. Major potential interactions with citalopram and venlafaxine.
Methylphenidate (Ritalin)	2.5 mg/d (start) Titrate up to 54 mg/d (27 mg D-isomer)	Schedule II. High-fat meals may increase AUC. Peak concentration 102 hours after ingestion. Do not use with MAOIs as it can precipitate hypertensive crisis. Antidepressants that increase norepinephrine can cause increased amphetamine side effects. Concomitant use with SSRI can result in increased SSRI concentrations.
Modafinil (Provigil)	50–100 mg (start) 100–200 mg every morning	Schedule IV. Avoid driving/operation of machinery until effects are known. Do not take at bedtime. Peak concentration in 2–4 hours. Food slows absorption by about 1 hour but does not affect bioavailability. Decreases efficacy of birth control pills.
Armodifinil (Nuvigil)	50 mg (start) 25–250 mg every morning	Schedule IV. Avoid driving/operation of machinery until effects are known. Do not take at bedtime. Peak concentration in 2–4 hours. Food slows absorption by about 1 hour but does not affect bioavailability. Decreases efficacy of birth control pills.

AUC = Area under the curve; SSRI = selective serotonin uptake inhibitor.

imbalance and comorbidities may be optimized as indicated. Treatment for sleep dysfunction and comorbidities should be optimized; however, clinicians need to be aware of potential risks of sedative-hypnotics drugs causing daytime sleepiness, fatigue, and potential drug–drug interactions.

References

1. NCCN Clinical Practice Guidelines in Oncology. Cancer-related fatigue. Ver1. 2013. National Comprehensive Cancer Network [http://www.nccn.org/professionals/physician_gls/f_guidelines.asp#supportive]

2. Braun IM, Greenberg DB, Pirl WF. Evidenced-based report on the occurrence of fatigue in long-term cancer survivors. *J Natl Compr Canc Netw.* 2008 Apr;6(4):347–354.

3. Curt GA. The impact of fatigue on patients with cancer: overview of FATIGUE 1 and 2. *Oncologist.* 2000;5(Suppl 2):9–12.

4. Rao AV, Cohen HJ. Fatigue in older cancer patients: etiology, assessment, and treatment. *Semin Oncol.* 2008;35:633–642.

5. Giacalone A, Quitadamo D, Zanet E, Berretta M, Spina M, Tirelli U. Cancer-related fatigue in the elderly. *Support Care Cancer.* 2013;21(10):2899–2911.

6. Temel JS, Pirl WF, Recklitis CJ, Cashavelly B, Lynch TJ. Feasibility and validity of a one-item fatigue screen in a thoracic oncology clinic. *J Thorac Oncol.* 2006 Jun;1(5):454–459.

7. Mishra SI, Scherer RW, Snyder C, Geigle PM, Berlanstein DR, Topaloglu O. Exercise interventions on health-related quality of life for people with cancer during active treatment. Cochrane Database Syst Rev. 2012 Aug 15;8:CD008465.

8. Minton O, Richardson A, Sharpe M, et al.: Drug therapy for the management of cancer-related fatigue. Cochrane Database Syst Rev. 2010;7: CD006704.

9. U.S. Food and Drug Administration.: *FDA Drug Safety Communication: Erythropoiesis stimulating Agents (ESAs): Procrit, Epogen and Aranesp.* Silver Spring, MD: Author; 2010.

10. Rizzo JD, Brouwers M, Hurley P, et al. American Society of Clinical Oncology/American Society of Hematology clinical practice guideline update on the use of epoetin and darbepoetin in adult patients with cancer. *J Clin Oncol.* 2010;28(33):4996–5010.

11. Auret KA, Schug SA, Bremner AP, Bulsara M. A randomized, double-blind, placebo-controlled trial assessing the impact of dexamphetamine on fatigue in patients with advanced cancer. *J Pain Symptom Manage.* 2009;37(4):613–621.

12. Moss EL, Simpson JS, Pelletier G, Forsyth P. An open-label study of the effects of bupropion SR on fatigue, depression and quality of life of mixed-site cancer patients and their partners. *Psychooncology.* 2006;15(3):259–267.

Chapter 11

Pain

Roma Tickoo and Archana Bushan

Introduction

One out of every three patients treated for active cancer experiences pain, whereas more than three out of every four people with advanced disease will have pain.[1] Persistent pain significantly reduces the quality of life of cancer patients. In effect, 67 percent of all such patients describe the pain associated with cancer as distressing, 36 percent describe it as an unbearable aspect of the disease, and 32 percent describe the pain as being so bad that they wish to die.[2]

Pain interferes with sleep, appetite, and mood; it also contributes to anxiety and fatigue, negatively impacting dependence and tolerance. Concerns about pain are often misconstrued by patients, family members, and health-care providers. Barriers to pain management include fears of addiction both by health care providers, patients, and their caregivers.

This chapter uses the NCCN Clinical Practice Guidelines In Oncology (NCCN Guidelines®) for Adult Pain as a framework for a comprehensive approach to pain in the cancer patient.[3] See Tables 11.1–11.6.

Table 11.1 Pain Screening and Evaluation
One-Item, 0–10 Scale[3]
• "How much pain are you having, on a scale of 0 (no pain) to 10 (worst pain you can imagine)?" 0 = no pain 4–6 = moderate pain 1–3 = mild pain 7–10 = severe pain For a pain score of 5 or greater, re-evaluate or refer to a pain specialist.
Pain Assessment Tools
Over 100 validated instruments are available. Commonly used measures include:
• Brief Pain Inventory by Cleeland (eight-item questionnaire that assesses the presence, location, and severity of pain; interference caused by pain; and response pain treatment).[4]
• McGill Pain Questionnaire by Melzack (20-item questionnaire that assesses sensory, affective, and qualitative aspects of pain).[5]
• The Faces Pain Rating Scale (patients can point to the face that shows how much pain they are having).[6]
• The Pain Assessment in Advanced Dementia (PAINAD) scale (useful in patients who are unable to communicate their pain. Health-care workers can observe these 5 specific indicators: breathing, vocalization, facial expression, body language, and consolability).[7]

(continued)

Table 11.1 (Continued)

Comprehensive Pain Assessment[2]

- **Pain intensity:** How severe is the pain on the scale of 0–10?
- **Location** of the pain.
- **Quality** of the pain: Ask the patient to describe what the pain feels like.
  - **Somatic pain**: Arises from cutaneous or deep tissues. Described as aching, stabbing, throbbing or "pressure like" pain. Examples: pain from bony metastasis or postoperative pain.
  - **Visceral pain:** Arises from organ infiltration, compression, or stretching. Described as gnawing, cramping, aching, or sharp, depending on the location. May be referred to a cutaneous site such as diaphragmatic pain referred to shoulder.
  - **Neuropathic pain**: May occur from nerve infiltration, compression, or other damage. Described as sharp, tingling, burning, shooting akin to an electric shock or vise-like. Patients with diabetic or alcoholic neuropathy, herpes zoster, or cord compression can have neuropathic pain.

Cancer pain is often of mixed etiology or, if purely neuropathic, may be one of several pains experienced by a patient. For these reasons, opioids are used more frequently in patients with cancer-related neuropathic pain. Standard guidelines for the use of anticonvulsants (e.g. pregabalin (Lyrica®) and gabapentin (Neurontin®)), antidepressants (e.g. duloxetine (Cymbalta®) and tricyclic antidepressants), and topical treatments (e.g. capsaicin (Capzasin-P®) and lidocaine (Lidoderm®)) may be applicable, but there is a lack of good-quality clinical trials in cancer-related neuropathic pain. Choice is dictated not only by age, drug interactions, and comorbidities, but also by the coexistence of many symptoms in patients with cancer. Treating more than one symptom with a particular neuropathic pain agent can avoid polypharmacy.[8]

- **Pain history and descriptors**[3]
  - When did it start?
  - How long has it been present?
  - Has it changed in any way?
  - Is it intermittent or constant/continuous?
  - Do you have other symptoms?
  - Does the pain radiate or move anywhere?
  - What makes the pain worse? . . . better?
  - What has been tried to treat the pain? Has it helped? Are there side effects? What are the scheduled doses?
- **Etiology:** Underlying causes of the pain must be identified and treated when possible. Emergency problems like spinal cord compression or infection must be treated immediately.
- **Medical history:** Pain should be evaluated in the context of the cancer and other significant medical illnesses, as well as current medications including over-the-counter and complementary substances.
- **Psychosocial issues:** Evaluate for patient distress, cultural beliefs toward pain, family/caregiver support, psychiatric/substance abuse history, and patients' goal for comfort and function.
  - **Distress:** How much distress is the pain causing? Is the pain bearable or unbearable? Does the diffuseness of the distress suggest emotional suffering rather than nociception? What does the patient think that the pain means (e.g. tumor spread)? What are cultural, spiritual or religious concerns about pain?

(continued)

Table 11.1 (Continued)

- **Support:** Who does the patient have for support? Are family members or others available? Is anyone reliably helping to manage the pain and medications at home? Evaluate for polypharmacy and possible medication interactions/side effects.
  - *Goals and expectations*—Discuss patients' goals and expectations regarding pain management in the context of level of comfort and function. Include family/caregivers.
  - **Physical examination** with review of appropriate laboratory and imaging studies.
- **Psychiatric illness:** *Anxiety*—Conditioned anticipatory anxiety may begin before dressing changes or painful walking. Patients may seek analgesics to treat anxiety or insomnia rather than pain. *Depression*—When elderly patients have clinical depression, pain feels worse. They are more likely to have somatic complaints rather than mood complaints. Assess history of depression and current depressive symptoms (sleep disturbance; loss of interest; guilt/hopelessness/helplessness; low energy; concentration difficulties; appetite changes; psychomotor retardation; suicidal ideation). Treat the depressive syndrome as appropriate. *Substance Abuse*—Patients with psychiatric or opiate abuse histories may require higher doses due to tolerance. Addictive behavior: Use caution in patients with a history of drug dependence or alcoholism. Use initial screening tool ORT (Opioid Risk Tool): a higher risk score correlates with an increased likelihood of drug abuse.[9]

Risk Factors for Undertreatment[2]

- The cognitively impaired, the elderly, women, and minorities.
- Patients underreporting their pain.
- Language/communication and cultural barriers.
- History of substance abuse, psychiatric illness, neuropathic pain.
- Fear by physician of complications/overdosing patient/lack of training in pain management.
- Fear by patient to "become an addict," or be labeled as one.[10]

Table 11.2 Initial Treatment

Definitions[2]:	• *"Opioid Naïve"*—described as patients who are NOT chronically receiving opioid analgesics on a daily basis and, therefore, have not developed significant tolerance.
	(The FDA identifies tolerance as receiving at least 60 mg of morphine daily; at least 30 mg of oral oxycodone daily; or at least 8 mg of oral hydromorphone (Dilaudid®) daily or an equianalgesic dose of another opioid for a week or longer.)
	• *"Opioid Tolerant"*—includes patients who are chronically receiving an opioid analgesic on a daily basis.
	What is a 'rescue dose' or demand dose?—Patients with chronic persistent pain that is controlled on stable doses of long acting opioid should have provision of short acting medications to manage breakthrough or transient exacerbations in pain. The rescue dose is usually equivalent to 10–20% of the total daily dose and can be given every hour as needed. In usual practice this is offered every 3–4 hours as needed.

(continued)

Table 11.2 (Continued)

Overview	• The route of administration of opioid—oral versus intravenous—is based upon what is best suited for a patient's ongoing analgesic needs. • Screen for pain at each visit with the one instrument and the 0–10 scale. • If the pain score is greater than 0, evaluate with the comprehensive pain assessment. • Goal is to treat/diagnose underlying causes of the pain while providing analgesia. Individualize treatment to patient's wishes, with the goal of maximizing function and quality of life. • Initiate pain medications based on opioid tolerance and intensity of the pain.
Treatment	• **Mild pain** (score 1–3): Consider NSAID or acetaminophen (Tylenol®) without opioids if patient is not on analgesics. If pain is not relieved, consider slow titration of short-acting opioids. • **Moderate Pain** (score 4–6): Administer 5–10 mg of oral immediate-release morphine sulfate or equivalent and reassess in 4 hours. If the pain score has decreased by less than 50%, increase the dose by 25–50% and repeat assessment in 4 hours. If the pain score decreased by at least 50%, this is the "effective 4 hour dose." Give the effective dose every 4 hours as needed. • **Severe pain** (score 7–10): Rapidly titrate short-acting opioids. Administer 5–10 mg of oral immediate-release morphine sulfate and reassess after 60 minutes. If pain is unchanged, double the dose and repeat until pain score decreases by at least 50%; re-evaluate frequently. If pain score decreases by less than 50%, repeat the same dose and reassess. After pain score is decreased by at least 50%, calculate the total amount given over 4 hours for the "effective 4-hour dose."
Opioid Tolerant Patients	If experiencing breakthrough pain of intensity greater than or equal to 4, or a pain intensity less than 4 but goals of pain control are not being met → Continue long acting, and… • Calculate the previous 24-hour total oral or IV opioid requirement, and take 10–20% of that for calculation of new rescue dose. • Efficacy and adverse effects should be assessed every 60 minutes for oral opioids, and every 15 minutes for intravenous opioids. • On reassessment, if pain score remains unchanged or increased → administer 50–100% of previous rescue dose. Repeat at 60 minute intervals (for oral meds) or every 15 minutes (for IV meds). If pain score remains unchanged upon reassessment after 2–3 cycles of the opioid, then consider changing route of administration or alternate strategies. • Once pain score decreases to <4 → the current effective dose of either oral or intravenous can be administered "as needed" over initial 24 hours. • Ultimately, you will need to increase both around-the-clock and as-needed doses based on the intensity of the pain.

Table 11.3 Next Steps

Conversion to Longer- Acting Opioids[2]	• Once pain is stable on immediate-release opioids, consider switching to longer-acting opioids.
	• Calculate dose based on 24-hour requirement and prescribe equivalent dose of extended-release morphine sulfate (MS Contin®), extended release oxycodone hydrochloride (OxyContin®), or transdermal fentanyl (Duragesic®).
	• Provide rescue doses of short-acting opioids for breakthrough pain. Use immediate-release forms of the long-acting opioid whenever possible and allow rescue doses of 10–20% of the total 24-hour dosage every one hour as needed.
Managing side effects[2]	• Opioid related side effects include constipation, nausea, and vomiting, drowsiness, sedation, confusion, respiratory depression and hypotension.
	• Older patients are more sensitive to these side effects (especially constipation and delirium).
	• The narcotic may accumulate, depending upon its half-life, drug interactions, or inability to metabolize adequately. Doses should be reduced gradually if the cause of pain has been treated or if the patient has adequate pain relief.
	• Administer prophylactic bowel regimen for all patients; and antiemetics if nausea present.
	• Monitor and adjust medications for sedation and delirium. Opioids at higher doses increase the risk of delirium. Concomitant benzodiazepines raise the risk of delirium.
	• To reduce the risk of delirium, increase narcotics slowly, e.g., 25–50%, then decrease as tolerated to diminish problems with cognition and delirium.
	Use psychotropic medications to augment narcotics, e.g., neuroleptics for anxiety or cognitive impairment such as haloperidol (Haldol®) or quetiapine (Seroquel®); stimulants for alertness such as methylphenidate (Ritalin®), dextroamphetamine (Dexedrine®), and modafinil (Provigil®). However, these must be added with caution and with the awareness of the burden of polypharmacy and accumulation of side effects and drug interactions.
Special Pain Issues[2]	• Pain related to oncologic emergency: Proceed *immediately* with treatment of the underlying condition in conjunction with pain medications.
	• **Bone pain:** In addition to trials of NSAIDS and/or opioids, other interventions are available for bone pain.
	• If pain is diffuse → Can use bisphosphonates, hormonal therapies (such as androgen deprivation therapy in prostate cancer or chemotherapy for responsive tumors, glucocorticoids, and/or systemic administration of radioisotopes is beneficial.

(continued)

Table 11.3 (Continued)

	• If the pain is localized → consider local radiation therapy or nerve block. For resistant pain, consider referral to anesthesia, orthopedics, or neurosurgery. • **Neuropathic pain:** Can use adjuvant analgesics such as anticonvulsants (i.e., pregabalin (Lyrica®) and gabapentin (Neurontin®)), anti-depressants (i.e., SNRI's, tricyclic antidepressants), corticosteroids, and local anesthetics/topical agents (i.e., topical lidocaine patch (Lidoderm®) or diclofenac gel (Voltaren gel®)). • **Pain from inflammation:** Pain from inflammation may be best treated by decreasing the inflammation with NSAIDS or glucocorticoids. **Nerve compression or inflammation**: A trial of glucocorticoids is indicated. • Also, prior to the use of NSAIDs→ rule out recent history of a GI bleed, renal impairment, low platelet count, active use of anticoagulation and steroids. • If pain is not adequately controlled by analgesics, or if the side effects have become intolerable, a referral to anesthesia or neurosurgery for a pain relieving procedure (i.e., nerve block) may be indicated
Non-pharmacological Modalities[2]	• Since pain encompasses physical, cognitive, and spiritual dimensions, having a comprehensive treatment approach is necessary. • Physical modalities include heat or ice; ultrasonic stimulation; transcutaneous electrical nerve stimulation (TENS); acupuncture, and massage. Physical therapy consultation might be useful for better positioning; strengthening compensatory muscle groups; and supplying bed, bath, and walking supports. • Cognitive interventions include: breathing exercises, relaxation techniques, imagery/hypnosis, distraction, and other behavioral therapies can be helpful. • Emotional support and education for the patient and family is essential. • A referral to a psychiatrist, psychologist, or social worker may be particularly helpful in evaluating and treating mood and anxiety symptoms related to the pain, delirium, sedation, and other mental status changes.

Adapted from Breivik H, Cherny N, Collett B, et al. Cancer-related pain: a pan-European survey of prevalence, treatment, and patient attitudes. *Ann Oncol.* Aug 2009;20(8):1420–1433.

Table 11.4 Opioid Medications

Opioid*	Parenteral	Oral Dose	Duration of Action
Morphine	10 mg	30 mg	3–4 hours
Hydromorphone (Dilaudid®)	1.5 mg	7.5 mg	2–3 hours
Levorphanol (Levo-Dromoran®)	2 mg	4 mg	3–6 hours
Oxycodone	—	15–20 mg	3–5 hours
Hydrocodone	—	30–45 mg	3–5 hours
Oxymorphone (Opana®)	1 mg	10 mg	3–6 hours
Codeine	—	200 mg	3–4 hours
Fentanyl (Duragesic®)	See below		
Methadone-	Consult Pain or Palliative Care Specialist if unfamiliar with methadone prescribing, as conversion ratios can vary.		

*In a single-dose administration, 10 mg IV morphine is equivalent to approximately 100 mcg IV fentanyl but with chronic fentanyl administration, the ratio of 10 mg IV morphine is equivalent to approximately 250 mcg of IV fentanyl. Based on this, in an opioid tolerant patient with chronic pain, we would consider 1 mg of IV Morphine sulfate equal to 25 mcg of Fentanyl IV and or Transdermal Patch/hourly.

*Continuous parenteral infusion fentanyl: transdermal fentanyl has a 1:1 ratio.

* Duration of fentanyl patch analgesic is usually 72 hours, but some patients may require patch replacement every 48 hours.

Table 11.5 NonOpioid Analgesics

Medication	Usual Dose	Side Effects
Ibuprofen (Advil®, Motrin®)	400 mg four times a day (maximum daily dose = 3,200 mg)	Epigastric pain; gastric or duodenal ulcers; GI bleeding; tinnitus; nausea and vomiting; nervousness; rash. Use caution in patients at high risk for renal, GI, or cardiac toxicities; thrombocytopenia, or bleeding disorders.
Ketorolac (Toradol®)	15–30 mg IV Q 6 hours for maximum of 5 days	Same as previous
Choline and magnesium salicylate combinations	1.5–4.5 g in 3 divided doses	Same as previous
Salsalate (Salflex®)	2–3 g in 2 or 3 divided doses	Nausea; GI bleeding; tinnitus; hearing impairment; hepatic dysfunction; decreased creatinine clearance
Acetaminophen (Tylenol®)	650 mg q 4 hr (maximum daily dose = 4 g)	Hepatic dysfunction; hepatic failure; renal disease; nephropathy; anemia; SIADH; transient hypothermia

Table 11.6 Medications for Neuropathic Pain

Medication	Starting Dosage	Titration	Maximum Dosage	Duration of Adequate Trial	Major Side Effects	Precautions	Other Benefits
Nortriptyline (Pamelor®) Desipramine (Norpramin®)	25 mg at bedtime	Increase by 25 mg daily every 3–7 days, as tolerated until pain relief	150 mg daily	6-8 weeks with >2 week at maximum tolerated dosage	Sedation, dry mouth, blurred vision, weight gain, urinary retention, orthostatic hypotension	Cardiac disease, glaucoma, suicide risk, seizure disorder, concomitant use of tramadol	Improvement of depression, insomnia, low cost. *Least anticholinergic effect, orthostatic hypotension and sedation. [11]
Duloxetine (Cymbalta®)	30 mg once daily	Increase to 60 mg once daily after 1 week	60 mg twice daily	4 weeks	Nausea	Hepatic dysfunction, renal insufficiency, alcohol abuse, concurrent use with tramadol	Improvement of depression
Venlafaxine (Effexor®)	37.5 mg once or twice daily	Increase by 75 mg each week, as tolerated until pain relief	225 mg daily	4–6 weeks	Nausea	Concurrent use of tramadol, cardiac disease, withdrawal syndrome if abrupt discontinuation	Improvement of depression

Gabapentin (Neurontin®)	100–300 mg QHS or 100-300 mg TID	Increase by 100–300 mg TID very 1–7 days, as tolerated, until pain relief	3600 mg daily (1200 mg TID), reduce if renal impairment	3–8 weeks for titration PLUS 2 weeks at maximum dose	Sedation, dizziness, peripheral edema	Renal insufficiency	Improvement of sleep disturbance, anxiety
Pregabalin (Lyrica®)	50 mg TID or 75 mg BID	Increase to 300 mg daily after 3–7 days, then by 150 mg/day every 3–7 days, as tolerated, until pain relief	600 mg daily (200 mg TID or 300 mg BID), reduce if impaired renal function	4 weeks	Sedation, dizziness, peripheral edema	Renal insufficiency	Improvement of sleep disturbance, anxiety
5% Lidocaine Patch (Lidoderm®)	Maximum of 3 patches daily for maximum of 12 hours	None needed	Maximum of 3 patches daily for maximum of 12 hours	3 weeks	Local erythema, rash	None	No systemic side effects

Adapted from O'Connor AB, Dworkin RH. Treatment of neuropathic pain: an overview of recent guidelines. *Am J Med.* Oct 2009;122(Suppl 10):S22–32.

References

1. Margarit C, Julia J, Lopez R, et al. Breakthrough cancer pain—still a challenge. *Journal of Pain Research*. 2012;5:559–566.

2. Breivik H, Cherny N, Collett B, et al. Cancer-related pain: a pan-European survey of prevalence, treatment, and patient attitudes. *Ann Oncol*. Aug 2009;20 (8):1420–1433.

3. NCCN. Adult Cancer Pain Guidelines version 2.2013. http://www.nccn .org/professionals/physician_gls/f_guidelines.asp#supportive2013.

4. Cleeland CS, Ryan KM. Pain assessment: global use of the Brief Pain Inventory. *Ann Acad Med, Singapore*. Mar 1994;23(2):129–138.

5. Melzack R. The McGill Pain Questionnaire: major properties and scoring methods. *Pain*. Sep 1975;1(3):277–299.

6. O'Connor AB, Dworkin RH. Treatment of neuropathic pain: an overview of recent guidelines. *Am J Med*. Oct 2009;122(Suppl 10):S22–S32.

7. Warden V, Hurley AC, Volicer L. Development and psychometric evaluation of the Pain Assessment in Advanced Dementia (PAINAD) scale. *J Am Med Directors Assoc*. Jan-Feb 2003;4(1):9–15.

8. Fallon MT. Neuropathic pain in cancer. *Brit J anaesthes*. July 2013;111(1):105–111.

9. Chou R, Fanciullo GJ, Fine PG, Miaskowski C, Passik SD, Portenoy RK. Opioids for chronic noncancer pain: prediction and identification of aberrant drug-related behaviors: a review of the evidence for an American Pain Society and American Academy of Pain Medicine clinical practice guideline. *J Pain*. Feb 2009;10(2):131–146.

10. Periyakoil V. Persistent pain. In: Durso S, Sullivan G, eds. *Geriatrics Review Syllabus: A Core Curriculum in Geriatric Medicine*, 8th ed: New York: American Geriatrics Society; 2013: 129–139.

11. Monks R, Merskey H. Psychotropic drugs In: Melzack R, Wall P, eds. *Handbook of Pain Management: A Clinical Companion to the Textbook of Pain*, 4th ed. Philadelphia, USA: Churchill Livingstone; 2003: p365.

Chapter 12

Sexual Dysfunction

Mary K. Hughes, Stephanie Lacey, and Christian J. Nelson

Introduction

Sexuality is an important quality of life issue for everyone, regardless of age or health status. Many older adults are sexually active; approximately 53% of adults between the ages of 65 to 74 are sexually active, while 26% between the ages of 75 and 85 are still sexually active.[1] Sexuality and intimacy can be impacted by any type of cancer. Often the geriatric patient presents to cancer treatment with preexisting sexual dysfunction. Sexuality is one of the first elements of daily living disrupted by a cancer diagnosis and, unlike other side effects of cancer and its treatments, these problems do not tend to resolve after several years of disease-free survival.[2] Nurses tend to avoid asking older patients about sexual health especially if they are also older.[3]

Menopausal symptoms can be very distressing to women and interfere with sexuality because of the changes to their bodies.[4] These changes happen gradually in women without cancer, who have time to adjust and enjoy sexual activity five to ten years longer with fewer sexual problems than women with cancer who rapidly experience menopause.[5] Women in surgical menopause suffer from more sexual problems than women in natural menopause.[5] The most common sexual concerns of women of all ages include loss of sexual desire, problems with arousal, inability to achieve orgasm, painful intercourse, negative body image, and diminished sexual desirability and attractiveness.[6]

In men, the most common sexual concerns include erectile dysfunction (ED), difficulty reaching orgasm, dry orgasm, painful orgasm/ejaculation, orgasm associated urine leak, penile length alterations, penile curvature (Peyronie's Disease) and low sexual desire. These concerns may differ depending on the type of cancer and treatment, but may also occur in the absence of cancer, and can cause a significant amount of distress.

Addressing sexual issues demonstrates to the patient that the clinician is open to questions and concerns about sexuality. Using Annon's PLISSIT Model of sexual assessment,[7] the clinician can open the discussion about sexuality with the aid of open-ended questions (see Table 12.1).

Tables 12.5–12.5 outline phases of sexual function (Table 12.2), factors affecting sexual function (Table 12.3) treatment of sexual function (Table 12.4), and referral resources for sexual dysfunction (Table 12.5).

Table 12.1 Annon's PLISSIT Model

Permission	Give permission to talk and think about sexuality and cancer at the same time: "What changes have you noticed sexually?" "Sexually, how are things going?" "Tell me about any sexual changes." "How has this affected you sexually?"
Limited Information	Tell the patient about sexual side effects: Erectile dysfunction, alopecia, alibido, vaginal dryness, and menopausal symptoms.
Specific Suggestions	Make suggestions to help with sexual dysfunction (i.e., vaginal lubricants and moisturizers, medications, position changes, sensate focusing, safer sex).
Intensive Therapy	Refer to marital therapist, sexual therapist or psychotherapist.

Adapted from Annon JS. The PLISSIT model: a proposed conceptual scheme for the behavioral treatment of sexual problems. *Journal of Sex Education and Therapy.* 1976;2(2):1–15.[7]

Table 12.2 Phases of Sexual Function and Causes of Dysfunction

Phases—Description and Dysfunction	Causes of Dysfunction	
Libido—Instinctual; multi-determined process; urge for or interest in sexual intercourse; controlled by testosterone **Disinterest in sexual activity; absence of sexual fantasies and dreams**	• Anxiety • Body image • Chemotherapy • Depression • Fatigue • Hormones	• Medications • Menopause • Pain • Prostate cancer • Relationship changes
Arousal—Increase in heart rate, respiratory rate, blood pressure and pelvic blood volume; in women, vaginal lubrication and swelling of genital tissues; in men, penile erection **In women, vaginal dryness; in men, erectile dysfunction (consistent inability to obtain and/ or maintain an erection sufficient for satisfactory sexual insertion)**	• Anxiety • Body image • Chemotherapy • Depression • Dyspareunia • Fatigue • Medications including hormones	• Menopause • Neuropathies • Pain • Surgery for gynecological, prostate or rectal/anal cancers • Radiation to pelvic area
Orgasm—Rhythmic contraction of smooth muscles in and around the genitals; sense of physical pleasure and release; in men, ejaculation **Delayed; absent; happens too quickly; retrograde or dry ejaculation**	• Anxiety • Chemotherapy • Depression • Fatigue • Medications	• Menopause • Pain • Radiation to pelvic area • Surgery to pelvic organs
Resolution—Period after orgasm; muscles relax, blood leaves genitals; penis flaccid, vaginal lubrication ends *Refractory period*—Length of time for the penis to "reset" and another erection to be possible **Refractory period lasting a day or more**	• Anxiety • Depression • Medications • Surgery	

Adapted from Hughes M. Disorders of sexuality and reproduction. In: Berger AM SJ, VonRoenn JH, ed. *Principles and Practice of Palliative Care and Supportive Oncology.* 4th ed.[8]

Table 12.3 Factors Affecting Sexual Function

Physical Changes	• Alopecia • Amputation • Anemia • Central nervous system changes • Fatigue • Hormone imbalances • Immunosuppression • Incontinence • Insomnia	• Ostomy • Pain • Menopausal symptoms • Muscle atrophy • Shortness of breath • Scars • Sterility • Thrombocytopenia • Weight changes
Nutritional disturbances affecting ability for and interest in kissing and being touched	• Anorexia • Constipation • Diarrhea • Dry mouth • Mucositis	• Nausea • Vomiting • Taste alterations associated with treatment
Psychological factors	• Adopting the 'patient' role (asexual) • Altered body image • Feelings of anxiety, depression and anger • Fears of death, rejection by partner, loss of control	• Guilt regarding behavior imagined as the cause of a disease or disability • Reassignment of priorities
Social and interpersonal factors	• Communication difficulties regarding feelings or sexuality • Difficulty initiating sexual activity after a period of abstinence • Fear of being contagious	• Fear of physically damaging an ill or disabled partner • Lack of imagination • Lack of a partner • Lack of privacy

Adapted from Tierney DK. Sexuality: a quality-of-life issue for cancer survivors. *Seminars in oncology nursing.* May 2008;24(2):71–79.[9]

Table 12.4 Treatment of Sexual Dysfunction

Hypoactive Sexual Desire Disorder	• Medicate physical symptoms (pain, nausea, etc.) • Treat anxiety and depression or change antidepressants, e.g. bupropion (Wellbutrin®) • Refer to sexual therapist • Regular exercise • Shower together	• Testosterone supplement or refer to endocrinologist • Estrogen supplements (Estring® or vaginal estrogen cream) • L-arginine for women who cannot take estrogen (anecdotal) • Schedule sexual encounters • Erotica—books, movies

(continued)

Table 12.4 (Continued)

Female Sexual Interest/Arousal Disorder	• Water soluble vaginal lubricants • Vaginal moisturizers • Natural oils (coconut, almond, olive) • EROS-CTD®—a vacuum device for females • Vibrators	• Vaginal dilators • Positional change • Treat depression and anxiety • Sensate focus exercises • Masturbate
Erectile Disorder	• Oral medications (PDE5 inhibitors), e.g. sildenafil citrate (Viagra®), vardenafil (Levitra®), tadalafil (Cialis®) • Penile injections • Vacuum/constriction device • Suppositories • Penile implant (prostheses) • Psychoeducation	• Address anxiety, distress, depression, anger • Penile band • Vibrators • Positional change • Masturbate • Couple's therapy • Sensate focus exercises • Individual counseling
Female Orgasmic Disorder	• Change antidepressants (SSRIs can delay orgasm; consider substituting bupropion (Wellbutrin®) • Vibrators • Masturbate	• Positional change • Refer to sexual therapist • Psychostimulants, e.g. modafinil (Provigil®), methylphenidate (Ritalin®), armodafinil (Nuvigil®) • Sensate focus exercises

Genito-Pelvic Pain/Penetration Disorder (Dyspareunia/ Vaginismus)	• Dilators in conjunction with Kegel exercises
	• Long-acting non-hormonal moisturizers
	• Lubricants
	• Referral to pelvic floor physical therapist
		• Low-dose local estrogen therapy (may be contraindicated)
		  • Estradiol vaginal cream (Estrace®)
		  • Conjugated estrogen vaginal cream (Premarin®)
		  • Sustained release silastic ring that releases estradiol (Estring®)
		  • Micronized estradiol hemihydrate vaginal pill (Vagifem®)

Adapted from Hughes M. Disorders of sexuality and reproduction. In: Berger AM SJ, VonRoenn JH, ed. *Principles and Practice of Palliative Care and Supportive Oncology*. 4th ed.[8]

DeVita VT LT, Rosenberg SA, ed *DeVita, Hellman, and Rosenberg's Cancer: Principles & Practice of Oncology*. 8th ed. Philadelphia: Lippincott Williams & Wilkins; 2009; No. 2.[10]

Table 12.5 Referral Resources for Sexual Dysfunction

Referrals	Reason
Bowel management specialist	Diarrhea; constipation
Cardiologist	Assess cardiac function for PDE5 inhibitors
Endocrinologist	Hormone, thyroid replacement; fertility issues
Fatigue specialist	Manage fatigue
Marital therapist[32]	Marital issues
Nutritionist, dietitian	Weight control, loss; bowel problems; nausea
Pain specialist	Pain control
Psychiatrist	Depression; anxiety; adjustment disorder
Psychologist, Advanced Practice Nurse	Behavioral, psycho-education, supportive therapy
Reproductive specialist	Fertility issues
Social worker	Housing; therapy
Sexual therapist	Sexual therapy, www.aasect.org, www.therapistlocator.net

References

1. Lindau ST, Schumm LP, Laumann EO, Levinson W, O'Muircheartaigh CA, Waite LJ. A study of sexuality and health among older adults in the United States. *N Engl J Med.* Aug 23 2007;357(8):762–774.

2. Schover LR. Premature ovarian failure and its consequences: vasomotor symptoms, sexuality, and fertility. *J Clin Oncol.* Feb 10 2008;26(5):753–758.

3. Hellwig J. Birth Trends: changes observed over a half century. *Nursing for women's health.* 2012;16(3):192–197.

4. Hughes MK. Alterations of sexual function in women with cancer. *Seminars in oncology nursing.* May 2008;24(2):91–101.

5. Eden KJ, Wylie KR. Quality of sexual life and menopause. *Women's health.* Jul 2009;5(4):385–396.

6. Derogatis LR, Burnett AL. The epidemiology of sexual dysfunctions. *J Sex Med.* Feb 2008;5(2):289–300.

7. Annon JS. The PLISSIT model: a proposed conceptual scheme for the behavioral treatment of sexual problems. *Journal of Sex Education and Therapy.* 1976;2(2):1–15.

8. Hughes M. Disorders of sexuality and reproduction. In: Berger AM SJ, VonRoenn JH, ed. *Principles and Practice of Palliative Care and Supportive Oncology.* 4th ed. Philadelphia: Lippincott, Williams & Wilkins; 2013:663–673.

9. Tierney DK. Sexuality: a quality-of-life issue for cancer survivors. *Seminars in oncology nursing.* May 2008;24(2):71–79.

10. DeVita VT LT, Rosenberg SA, ed *DeVita, Hellman, and Rosenberg's Cancer: Principles & Practice of Oncology.* 8th ed. Philadelphia: Lippincott Williams & Wilkins; 2009; No. 2.

Special Considerations in Psychosocial Issues in Older Patients with Cancer

Chapter 13

Communicating with Older Cancer Patients

Elizabeth Harvey and Christian J. Nelson

Introduction

The communication between medical staff and an elderly patient can present a number of unique challenges. Some of these challenges are obvious. Deficits in hearing or sight can add frustration in the communication process for both the staff and the older patient. Other challenges are more subtle. Medical professionals often do not realize the impact ageism can have on care they provide and the communication they have with older adults. Older adults, as compared to medical professionals, may also have a different view on judging the balance between aggressive treatment vs. quality of life. Often times the treatment team assumes a patient would like the most advanced care. The older adult may be evaluating the treatment choice through a different perspective on life. A perspective that may include shorter time horizons, and as a result, the older adult may be more inclined to select a less aggressive treatment that preserves quality of life. This chapter outlines the issues and strategies to help address the complicated factors involved in working with elderly individuals.

There are specific issues involved in geriatric communication, including (See Adelman and Greene[1] for an expanded discussion of the topics listed below):

- Treatment discussion (Box 13.1)
- Ageism (Boxes 13.2–13.3)
- Sensory deficits (Boxes 13.4–13.5)
- Functional limitations (Box 13.6)
- Involving caregivers (Box 13.7)
- Mild cognitive impairment (Box 13.8)

Box 13.1 Treatment Discussion with Older Patients

- Do not assume the older patient would like the most aggressive treatment.
- Explore the older adult's current values and how these might influence treatment choice.
- Present treatment options.
- Take breaks in the communication, and have the patient paraphrase important aspects of the discussion.

Box 13.2 Ageism and Staff Interaction with Patients

- Staff members may disregard medical problems of older patients, attributing symptoms to aging. As a result, patients may not get the care they need.
- Staff members spend less time with geriatric patients and are less attentive to their concerns.
- Elderly patients are seen as "more difficult".
- Fear of one's own aging results in discrimination toward patients.
- It is hard to communicate with older patients amidst multiple physical problems, creating a limitation in staff ability to connect with these individuals.

Box 13.3 Strategies to Reduce/Combat Ageism

- The perspective of patients must be taken in to account to reduce stereotyping.
- Each patient must be seen as an individual, and the heterogeneity amongst older patients must be understood.
- It is important for professionals to learn more about their patients through active listening and life reviews.
- Staff members must create a safe environment for older cancer patients, providing opportunity and encouragement to introduce their concerns, and be engaged in the interaction.
- Psychosocial issues should be integrated into medical decision-making. Patients should feel comfortable discussing issues such as loneliness, anxiety, depression, and neglect. Physicians do not need to personally handle these issues, but they must be available to listen, to be emotional supportive, and to refer to the appropriate clinician if necessary.

Box 13.4 Hearing Strategies

- Good visual contact must be established.
- Reduce background noise where possible.
- Staff members should rephrase rather than repeat misunderstood phrases.
- Pausing at the end of a topic may help understanding.
- Professionals should stand or sit a few feet away from the patient, speaking slowly and slightly more loudly.
- Physicians should discuss and ask patients' opinion on the best way to communicate.
- In order to insure understanding, patients should be asked to repeat their understanding.

Box 13.5 Vision Strategies

- Staff members must sit close to the patient.
- Improve lighting where possible.
- Provide larger print materials.

Box 13.6 Functional Deficits

- The physical limitations of elderly patients may make the logistics of the visit difficult, for example handling a walker or a wheel chair.
- Frail patients who do not visit their doctor often may find the experience emotionally and physically taxing.
- Functional deficits may prolong the visit.
- Functional deficits require additional preplanning to accommodate patients.

Box 13.7 Involving Caregivers

- Professionals working with older patients frequently interact with family members/caregivers who accompany patients to their visits. Caregivers are often extremely involved in geriatric medical care, and staff members must find ways to include these individuals in order to meet patients' needs.
- Be aware that the caregivers and the patient may have different treatment goals.
- Talk to the patient first, and then the caregivers. Often times, older patients complain that the medical professional talks to the caregiver instead of the older adult.
- It may be beneficial to have professionals first meet with patients alone, and then invite caregivers to join the visit.

Box 13.8 Cognitive Impairment Strategies

- An accurate assessment of patients' cognitive status must be obtained for effective communication.
- Physicians must not generalize that patients with any degree of cognitive impairment are incapable of contributing to their own care.

Reference

1. Adelman RD, Greene MG, Ory, MG. "Communication Between Older Patients and Their Physicians." *Clin Geriat Med.* 2000;16(1):1–24.

Chapter 14

Demoralization, Despair, and Existential Concerns

Talia Weiss Wiesel

Older adults, especially those facing more urgent end-of-life issues, face a range of existential concerns, particularly demoralization[1]. Demoralization refers to a sense of regret over the life one has lived as well as a feeling of hopelessness.

Kissane describes demoralization as[2,3]:

- Existential despair.
- Hopelessness.
- Helplessness and personal failure.
- Subjective incompetence.
- Loss of meaning and purpose in life.
- Social alienation.
- Different from depression because there is as a sense of subjective failure to achieve life's goals.

In older patients[4]:

- Despair and angst associated with loss of purpose and meaning to life.
- Loss of relationships.
- Loss of some sense of who one is.
- These patients typically state, "I can't see the point anymore; there's no reason to go on."

Factors contributing to the development of demoralization[4,5]:

- Social isolation.
- Declining physical health.
- Disfigurement.
- Disability (e.g., deafness).
- Dependency.
- Perceived loss of dignity.
- Concern about being burden to family.
- Increased number of physical problems.*

In a prospective study of advanced cancer patients of all ages, Jacobsen[1] found it is associated with the patients' degree of inner peacefulness.

* Results regarding age, gender, and treatment phase are inconsistent.

Research from patients receiving palliative care and those near the end of life,[6] found that 14 percent report they are "demoralized." There is little research specifically focused on older patients with cancer who are struggling with existential distress.[7] A study looking at changes in and predictors of quality of life in older patients with cancer over time found they are in a vulnerable situation, and have problems in coping with existential issues 6 months after diagnosis.[8] The most vulnerable groups within this population included those with advanced disease and decreased hope. For many patients, hope and sense of worth is contingent on the ability to find continued meaning in their day-to-day existence.[9] The prevalence of demoralization occurring in the elderly has been shown to be double the rate of depression.[4] An intervention for distressed older adults (≥ aged 70 and older) with cancer showed a reduction in demoralization (as well as depression, anxiety, and loneliness). Patients also had an increase in spiritual well-being.[10]

References

1. Jacobsen J, Vanderwerker L, Block S, et al: Depression and demoralization as distinct syndromes: Preliminary data from a cohort of advanced cancer patients. *Indian J Palliat Care*. 2006;12:8–15.

2. Kissane DW, Love A, Hatton A, et al: Effect of cognitive-existential group therapy on survival in early stage breast cancer. *J Clin Oncol*. 2001;22:4255–4260.

3. Clarke DM, Kissane DW: Demoralization: Its phenomenology and importance. *Aust N Z J Psychiat*. 2002;36:733–742.

4. Kissane D: Demoralization—A useful conceptualization of existential distress in the elderly. *Aus J Ageing*. 2001;20:110–111.

5. Vehling S, Oechsle K, Koch U, et al: Receiving palliative treatment moderates the effect of age and gender on demoralization in patients with cancer. *PLoS ONE* 8, 2013.

6. Chochinov H: Dignity and the essence of medicine: The A, B, C, and D of dignity conserving care. *BMJ*. 2007;335:184–187.

7. Meisner RC, Khin Khin E, Dorfman J, et al: A 60-year-old male with hairy-cell leukemia and existential distress. *Psychiat Ann*. 2012;42:138–141.

8. Esbensen, BA, Østerlind K, Hallberg IR: Quality of life of elderly persons with cancer: a 6-month follow-up. *Scand J Caring Sci*. 2007;21:178–190.

9. Fehring R, Miller J, Shaw C. Spiritual well being, religiosity, hope, depression and other mood states in elderly people coping with cancer. *Oncol Nurs Forum*. 1997;24:663–671.

10. Roth A, Napolitano S, Kenowitz J, et al: A psychoeducational intervention for older cancer patients—The cancer and aging: Reflections for elders (CARE) intervention. *Psycho-oncology (Chichester, England) (1057–9249)*, 2012;21(suppl.1):42.

Chapter 15

Caregiver Burden

Barbara A. Given

Understanding the family burden experience requires good communication with the cancer professional and the caregiver. We need to help the caregiver acquire skills to provide care and mobilize resources. Caregiver burden outcomes should be established and clinical practice guidelines used for management.

Recommendations for standards of care for caregiver burden

1. Caregiver burden should be identified, monitored and documented in all family caregivers and recorded in cancer patient records.
2. Caregiver should be screened for their ability to provide care and their level of distress.
3. Caregiver should be screened at appropriate intervals, clearly at each transition point: treatment, end of treatment, remission, recurrence, disease progression, and end of life.
4. Screening should identify the level and nature of the burden.
5. All caregivers should be screened for caregiver burden and asked specific questions about their health and caregiver strain.
6. Acknowledge the important role played by the caregiver in cancer care.
7. Educate patients and families about the disease and appropriate modifications that must be made day to day in the home environment because patient safety is a concern.
8. Evaluate caregiver coping strategies and encourage caregivers to care for themselves.
9. If caregivers have burden, then they need to be referred to their own primary-care provider.
10. Refer burdened caregivers to appropriate community services.
11. Discuss legal and financial issues and obtain appropriate help for caregivers and families.

See Tables 15.1–15.8.

Table 15.1 Overview of Caregiver Burden

Topic	Caregiver Burden—Description
Definition—Caregiver burden	A state in which an individual is experiencing physical, emotional, and/or financial strain in the process of caring for another, which can occur when care demands outweigh available resources.[1] The extent to which caregivers feels that their emotional or physical health, social life, and financial status have suffered as a result of caring for their relatives.[2] (Care demands include: function, comorbidity, polypharmacy, nutritional status, psychological status, and cognitive function.)
Prevalence	Prevalence of caregiver burden is difficult to know. Burden is often not identified by health-care professionals. Most patients will require caregiver support, and 20–30 percent of them will be burdened.
Impact	Caregiver burden is a response the caregivers of cancer patients report as a result of the demands and tasks of care, uncertainty of care, and complex care they provide. Caregivers report physical, emotional, social, and spiritual distress as a result of providing care that impacts their physical and emotional health.
	Caregivers of the geriatric population often have more problems due to their own aging (frailty) and their own multiple comorbidities.
Questions to ask to assess the caregiving situation	Check on ability to balance caregiving with other life demands.
	What are patient needs?
	Do family and friends help?
	What type of help would you like?
	Do family and friends visit?
	Do you have outside help?
	Do you feel burdened by the tasks?
	Do you feel stressed/strained by tasks?
	Are you afraid of the future? Has your own physical or mental health suffered?
	Do you feel prepared to provide care?
	Do you know where to get support to provide care?

Table 15.2 Burden Screening and Evaluation—At Each Diagnosis and Major Care Transitions

Topic	Assessment
A Burden Screening Tool should be selected if caregiver appears burdened or at risk for burden	Use the **Family Stress Thermometer**[3] to assess caregiver needs or a caregiver burden tool (see list below).
	What is your emotional response to providing care?
	Do you feel sad or depressed?
	Does caregiver have decision making capacity?
	Does caregiver have family or other support?
	What is the cognitive function?

(continued)

Table 15.2 (Continued)

Topic	Assessment
Use Validated Instruments	Caregiver Response[1]
	Zarit Burden Inventory[2]
	Care Giver Oncology Quality of Life Questionnaire[4]
	Appraisal of Caregiving Scale[5]
	Caregiver Strain Index[6]
	Oberst Caregiver Demands[7]

Table 15.3 Burden History

Topic	Assessment
Onset of Burden	When did caregiving start?
	When did you first notice distress/burden?
	How many hours of care do you provide each week?
	What are the tasks of care you are now assisting with?
	How did the burden change over time?
	(Transitions in Care: diagnosis, start of treatment, during active treatment, in recurrence and disease progression, end of life, survivorship, and palliative care)
	How are you doing?

Table 15.4 Care-related Activities

Topic	Assessment
Level of Caregiver Functioning (If the caregiver appears frail and has functional limitations, a comprehensive geriatric assessment should be completed).	Can the caregiver do own ADL and IADL? What is his/her functional ability?
	Does caregiver have evidence of geriatric syndromes?
	Can caregiver provide transportation?
	Can the caregiver hear and see well enough to be able to provide care?
	Would community or family support help the caregiver?
	What aspects of care are most burdensome?
	What are the most difficult components of care?
	Is the home environment safe?
	Does the caregiver have chronic health problems that interfere with providing care?
Related to Cancer Treatment	Are the patient's symptoms and side effects controlled? Or do they appear to be problems for caregiver?
	Who helps you with patient care?
	What tasks are bothersome or difficult?
	What care is needed by the patient?
	Does the caregiver have the capacity to understand the relevant information for patient care?
	Does the caregiver tell you relevant information about the patient's conditions?
	Quality of patient's care should be determined; is care being given and does patient appear cared for?
	Are side effects managed?
	Does the caregiver know how to manage the patient's side effects from cancer treatment?

Table 15.5 Distinguishing Burden from Depression

Signs of Depression	For two or more continuous weeks, determine moderate to severe (4 or higher statement of depression on 0–10 scale). Ask:
	Do you often feel sad, blue or depressed?
	(If caregiver endorses feeling sad or depressed administer the Geriatric Depression Scale).
	Are you unable to experience enjoyment or pleasure?
	Do you feel down hearted?
	Do you have a decreased interest in your surroundings?
	Are you unable to concentrate?
	Do you feel hopeless?
	Do you have a loss of energy?
	Are you fearful?
	Do you feel suicidal?
Signs of Burden	Feelings of distress and burden are due to the context of caring (affected by amount, duration) of care (if persistent may lead to depression). Ask:
	Do you feel you are not coping with providing care?
	Do you worry and are you anxious about the patient's care?
	Do you feel irritable about care?
	Do you feel strained by your care?
	Do you feel pressured or overwhelmed by the care/time?
	Do you have difficulties performing tasks?
	Are you worried about future demands of care?
	Do you feel stressed by the care *and* trying to meet your other responsibilities?
	Do you feel your relative is too dependent on you?
	Do you feel prepared to provide care?
	Do you feel providing care is confining?
	(Provider should determine preoccupation with care activities hypervigilance)

Table 15.6 Causes of Burden	
Topic	**Assessments**
Causes of Cancer Related Caregiver Burden	Number of patients' comorbidities
	Caregiver load, number of hours of care
	Physical dependency of patient (ADL and IADL limitations)
	Financial pressure from care
	Disruptive patient behaviors/behavioral problems
	Changes in care demands either increase or decrease
	Uncertainty in care expectations, fear for the future
	Severity and duration of patients' illness and care demands
	Caregivers' other competing role demands family and work
	Complexity of care (multisymptoms, procedures)
	Symptom burden of patient
Available Support	Ask the caregiver:
	What do you need help with?
	Who would help you with patient's care?
	Who helps now with patient care?
	Who would help you in an emergency or to get patient to a care center?

Table 15.7 Interventions	
Common Categories of Interventions for Caregivers with Burden	Cognitive behavioral interventions
	Psycho-educational interventions—help cope (education and information)
	Supportive interventions (social, family, community)
	Problem solving
	Multicomponent interventions (education problem solving, support counseling)
	Counseling—for managing stress and coping

Table 15.8 Indicators of Burden

Topic Area	Assessment	Consults or Referrals	Intervention
Indicators of Burden	• Frustration about care responsibilities • Reluctance to get help • Preoccupation with care activities/hypervigilant—enmeshed in the care • Competing roles—family and work) • Anger • Disturbed sleep • Irritability and impatience, anxious and worry • Feels abandoned by family • Feeling and expressing being overwhelmed and out of control • Apprehension about ability to providing "good" care • Uncertainty about future • Difficulty focusing on providing care and tasks, making decisions	Counselor, psychologist Refer caregiver to their own primary care physician or nurse practitioner	• Assessment—Systematic • Assessment for distress with Stress Thermometer or Burden Scale[1,2,4,8] • Re evaluate each transition • Help caregiver to reframe, to ask for assistance • Stress management techniques should be recommended • Provide support • Identify all sources of help and meet with support group (Consider the Wellness Community, online groups, Cancer Care, ACS) • Develop a coordinated plan • If appropriate use Survivorship Care Plan • What are expectations for patient's future? Be sure caregiver understands

Risk factors for negative outcomes	• Being a female • Other life stressors • Number of tasks complexity and patient deterioration or increased dependency • Caregiver may have their own physical disability • Communication issues between patient and caregiver • Anxiety and depression of caregiver • Lower socioeconomic status with financial problems • History of previous bad relationships/family conflicts • Lack of social support	Social worker, Financial planner Counselor Discharge planning Support group (in person or online)	• Obtain family support • Have a family meeting • Help caregiver develop communication skills to communicate with providers and other family members • Obtain social support • Ensure that caregivers are aware of community supports • Have them rehearse communication with professionals or family members • Help mobilize resources • Provide info to assist caregiver with responsibility of care • Acknowledge caregiver distress and burden
Response to Past Interventions for Burden or Distress	• What do caregivers do to get help? • Do you accept help when needed? • Previous treatment for depression (history of) • Relationships with caregiver • What do you do to relieve stress and tension or burden? • Have you tried recommendations by health professional to deal with burden? • Do they communicate concerns to providers?	Social worker Counselor	• Mobilize resources • Help them change meaning and expectations so they do not become hypervigelent • Recommend stress reduction approaches • Provide counseling—provide information to reduce uncertainty • Acknowledge caregiver burden • Relaxation, mindfulness, meditation and guided imagery

(continued)

Table 15.2 (Continued)

Topic Area	Assessment	Consults or Referrals	Intervention
Quality of Patient Care	• Is patient getting the care they need?: • For symptom control • To keep needed appointments • Other procedures • Inability to problem solve or make decisions • Caregiver lacking information to provide care	Meeting with nurse or Patient Educator Discharge planner Use of Home Care Patient education information from: ACS, NCI, COPE Wellness Community	• Determine outcomes to be achieved • Determine if they need help in coordinating patient care • Skill development/building for caregiver • Mobilize resources • Utilize problem solving using methods such as COPE[9] • Use Symptom Management Toolkit[10] to: • Guide families on how to manage patient symptoms. • Recommend respite sources • Telephone or web based counseling • Recommend decision AIDS • Home Management Guides[9] • Caregiver self care

| Caregiver Burden Management | • Use Caregiver Burden Assessment[1]
• Check about depression
• Caregiver concern about giving care in areas of difficulty or areas of distress | Primary care provider (Caregivers)
Social worker
Support groups
Counseling service
Minister or chaplain | • Use distress thermometer[3] for assessment of specific areas of distress areas of concern
• Monitor burden at each visit
• Acknowledge caregiver burden
• Mobilize resources and support
• Recommend stress management exercises and physical activity
• Provide needed information
• Obtain counseling referral
• Provide resource list
• Teach problem solving skills
• Telephone support from professional
• Telephone support from fellow caregivers
• Identify quality online support from fellow caregivers
• Respite services |

References

1. Given CW, Given B, Stommel M, Collins C, King S, Franklin S. The caregiver reaction assessment for caregivers to persons with chronic physical and mental impairments. *Res Nurs Health*. 1992;15(4):271–283.

2. Bedard M, Molloy DW, Squire L, Dubois S, Lever JA, O'Donnell, M. The Zarit burden interview: A new short version and screening version. *Gerontologist*. 2001;41(5):652–657.

3. van Dooren S, Duivenvoorden HJ, Passchier J, et al. The distress thermometer assessed in women at risk of developing hereditary breast cancer. *Psychooncol*. 2009;18(10):1080–1087.

4. Minaya P, Baumstarck K, Berbis J, et al. The caregiver oncology quality of life questionnaire (CarGOQoL): Development and validation of an instrument to measure the quality of life of the caregivers patients with cancer. *Eur J Cancer*. 2012;48(6):904–911.

5. Stetz K. The relationship among background characteristics, purpose in life, and caregiving demands on perceived health of spouse caregivers. *Sch Inq Nurs Pract*. 1989;3(2):133–153.

6. Robinson BC. Validation of a caregiver strain index. *J Gerontol* 1983;38(3):344–348.

7. Oberst MT, Thomas SE, Gass KA, Ward SE. Caregiving demands and appraisal of stress among family caregivers. *Cancer Nurs*. 1989;12(4):209–215.

8. Zarit SH, Reever KE, Bach-Peterson J. Relatives of the impaired elderly: Correlates of feelings of burden. *Gerontologist*. 1980;20(6):649–655.

9. Houts PS, Nezu AM, Nezu CM, Bucher JA. The prepared family caregiver: A problem-solving approach to family caregiver education. *Patient Educ Couns*. 1996;27(1):63–73.

10. Given BA, Given CW, Majeske C. *Symptom management toolkit*. East Lansing, MI: Michigan State University, 2012.

Further Reading

National Comprehenisve Cancer Network. NCCN Clinical Practice Guidelines in Oncology: Distress Management, (Version 2.2013). Fort Washington, PA: Author, 2013.

National Comprehenisve Cancer Network. NCCN Clinical Practice Guidelines in Oncology: Senior Adult Oncology, (Version 2.2013). Fort Washington, PA: Author, 2013.

Chapter 16

Advance Directives

Talia Weiss Wiesel and Yesne Alici

Definitions[1]

Advance directives (also referred to as *advance care directives*) are instructions outlined by patients that are intended to ensure that patients' wishes regarding end-of-life care are respected and carried out, even when the patients no longer have the capacity to make decisions for themselves. The advance directives came into being with the primary objective of protecting individual autonomy. The title by which it is referred to, the constituents of the document, and the procedure to prepare it vary by country or even states within the same country. It broadly consists of two components and may document an individual's wishes with respect to life-sustaining treatment (living will), their choice of a surrogate decision maker (durable power of attorney for health care) or both.

Advance care planning is the process in which patients, usually along with their families and health-care practitioners discuss and consider their values and goals for end-of-life care and formulate preferences for future care.

Written advance directives formalize the preferences of the patient and include:

- **Living will**: A living will describes the type of treatment and care the patient would like to receive and gives specific instructions about procedures (e.g., feeding tubes, mechanical ventilation) the patient would or would not like to prolong his/her life.
- **Durable power of attorney for health care**: The document that names the *health-care proxy* (also referred to as the surrogate decision maker), the person appointed the power by the patient to make health-care decisions when it has been determined that the patient cannot make such decisions his/herself.
- **"Do-Not-Resuscitate" (DNR) orders**: is written by physicians to operationalize the patient's/their proxy's preferences for the patient to not be resuscitated.

When to Initiate End-of-Life Care Discussions with Older Adults?

Clinicians may find it difficult to initiate end-of-life care discussions. This may lead to an unnecessary delay in allowing patients and families to discuss their goals and preferences. If a patient hasn't discussed advance care directives with his/her primary-care physician the current treating clinician should assume the responsibility and inquire about the patient's goals and preferences. Clinicians may bring up the subject when discussing prognosis, treatment options with a low likelihood of success, and patients' hopes and fears about the future. For patients facing imminent death, it is urgent to review a patient's goals and preferences for end-of-life care.[1]

When are advance directives most useful?

- When there is disagreement among family members.
- When there is conflict between the family and health-care team.
- When the patient assigns a nontraditional family member (e.g., friend or same sex partner) as the surrogate.[2,3]

1. Prepare the patient and the family members for the discussion:

Before meeting with the patient about advance directives, the clinician should have a good understanding of the patient's medical condition and prognosis. The clinician should review what is known about the patient's goals and values, and the patient's capacity to make end-of-life care decisions. The family members involved in the patient's care should be determined or found out about before the meeting. An uninterrupted time for discussion should be scheduled.

2. Establish trust with the patient and the family:

Patients and families should be encouraged to talk about what they know about the patient's condition and prognosis. Any misunderstandings about the illness or the prognosis should be clarified. The clinician should demonstrate respect to patients and families, and stay away from forcing any decisions on them. If the patient or the family members need more time to make a decision they should be allowed to present a decision when they are ready.

3. Be empathic to the patient's and the family's affects:

The clinician should acknowledge the emotions as they appear during the advance care directives discussion, and he or she should validate and explore the patient and the family's feelings. It is also important for clinicians to reinforce commitment to the patient and family at all stages of the illness through the end of life.

4. Foster hope in communicating treatment options:

Clinicians should help patients reframe hope by encouraging focus on short-term goals, symptom control, relief of suffering, and preparing for the worst while continuing to hope for the best.

Examples of questions to begin a conversation about advance care planning:[3]

- What are the biggest concerns you have about your illness?
- Thinking about your illness, what are the best and worst possible outcomes?
- Thinking about your illness, what has been most difficult or challenging for you?
- What are your expectations, hopes, and fears for the future?
- Thinking about the future, what matters most to you?

Examples of questions to clarify treatment preferences:[4]

- What can you tell me about the history of your illness?
- What do you understand about your treatment options?
- In terms of treatment, what are you worried about or afraid of?
- If a family member or loved one has died, how did they die, and what was that like for you?
- What are the practical problems associated with your illness?

Main motivations of older cancer patients to complete advance directives[5] (Pautex S, Notaridis G et al. 2010):

- To enhance autonomy.
- To enhance communication with caregivers.
- Fear of unnecessary or aggressive treatments.
- To reduce feeling like a burden to family members.
- To enhance communication with their surrogates.
- To be sure their preferences will be respected.

Assessment of Decision-Making Capacity

An important step before implementing surrogate decision makers, health care proxies or health-care power attorneys is to assess the patient's decision making capacity. The four pillars of decision-making capacity are understanding, appreciation, reasoning, and expressing a choice. Although cognitive impairment impacts one's ability to understand and express, it does not automatically preclude intact capacity. Any attending physician could determine a patient's decision-making capacity. In complex cases, psychiatry and/or ethics consultations could be sought for.

If a patient lacks capacity and the applicability of an advance directive is dubious, surrogate decision making may be considered in determining an accurate reflection of the patient's wishes. There are two approaches to surrogate decision making, namely the "substituted judgment" and "best interest." The "substituted judgment" principle is based on a patient's known values and the surrogate is required to make a decision based on their knowledge of the same. The "best interest" principle requires a surrogate to make a decision based on what would best serve the patient's interest and well-being.

References

1. McPhee SJ, Winkler MA, Rabow MW, et al. *JAMA Care at the Close of Life: Evidence and Experience*. American Medical Association, McGraw Hill; 2011.

2. Tulsky JA. Chapter 2. Beyond advance directives: importance of communication skills for care at the end of life. In: McPhee SJ, Winker MA, Rabow MW, Pantilat SZ, Markowitz AJ, eds. *Care at the Close of Life: Evidence and Experience*. New York, NY: McGraw-Hill; 2011.

3. Bomba PA, Kemp M, Black JS. POLST: An improvement over traditional advance directives. *Cleve Clin J Med*. 2012. 79(7):457–464.

4. Leland J. Advance directives and establishing the goals of care. *Primary Care*. 2001;28(2):349–363.

5. Pautex S, Notaridis G, Déramé L, Zulian GB. Preferences of elderly cancer patients in their advance directives. *Critical Rev Oncol/Hematol*. 2010;74(1):61–65.

Chapter 17

Psychosocial Issues in Elderly Minority Population

Talia Weiss Wiesel and Mark I. Weinberger

Introduction

The U.S. population is growing older and becoming more ethnically diverse.[1] Although non-Hispanic Whites account for the majority of the population (69%), the Hispanic and African American populations are growing faster than the population as a whole.[1] By the year 2030, it is projected that the elderly will account for 20 percent of the population, almost double the rate in 2005.[1] By 2050 there is an expected 99 percent increase in the incidence of cancer in in Blacks and Hispanics compared to a 31 percent increase in cancer incidence in Caucasians.[1] Older, ethnically diverse cancer patients will carry over a quarter (28%) of all cancer diagnoses.[1]

Psychosocial Service Needs in Ethnically Diverse Cancer Patients

Distress is significantly correlated with psychosocial needs in cancer patients and ethnically diverse cancer patients. Researchers have found 71 percent of ethnically diverse, underserved cancer patients who experienced clinically significant distress also endorsed psychosocial needs (i.e., provided contact information and a desire to be contacted regarding psychosocial services).[2] Areas of need include emotional, psychological, and social support; information; spiritual; sexual; financial and employment.[3]

Psychological Distress

Distress in Older Cancer Minority Patients

A 2010 study by Nelson et al. documented rates of distress, depression, anxiety, and well-being in older African American men with prostate cancer; in the nonmatched comparison, African American men had elevated levels of distress, anxiety, and depression similar to Caucasian men.[4] After matching the African-American and Caucasian men, African-American men reported significantly higher mean scores on emotional well-being and a significantly lower percentage of African American men displayed clinically significant depressive symptoms compared with Caucasian men

(4% versus 15%). After matching the sample, African American men seem to display a sense of resilience, demonstrating greater emotional well-being and a lower incidence of clinically significant depressive symptoms, compared with Caucasian men. This underscores the complexity of understanding the relationship between race and psychological distress.

Psychosocial Service Needs

Psychosocial Needs of Older Black and Hispanic Cancer Patients

Black and Hispanic oncology patients of all ages report more unmet needs than Caucasian patients.[5] There is little literature documenting the needs of ethnically diverse geriatric oncology patients. In a paper discussing ethnic and racial disparities in cancer care, Gansler et al. reported that "minority status" (race and ethnicity), individuals with less education, and the elderly are less likely to take advantage of health care services.[6]

Geriatric patients are often less satisfied with their care and less likely to express their needs than younger patients. Minorities are less likely to voice their needs and utilize psychosocial services than Caucasians. Taken together, we believe Black and Hispanic geriatric patients would be the group with the *highest need*, but are the *least likely* to utilize mental health services during or after their cancer treatment.

Barriers and Protective Factors in Older Black and Hispanic Patients

Research indicates Black and Hispanic geriatric oncology patients may face multiple potential barriers to receiving medical and psychosocial care. These barriers are related to ageism,[7] socioeconomic disparities,[8] health literacy,[9] and cultural/linguistic barriers.[10] Certain barriers (e.g., financial strain,[11] difficulty navigating the health-care system,[12] and underutilization of mental health services[12]) may contribute to greater levels of psychological distress. See Table 17.1.

Table 17.1 Barriers Regarding Psychological Distress among Ethnic Minority Cancer Patients	
Barriers in Older Patients:	Reduced hearing, vision, mobility
	Reduced social support
	Ageism
Barriers in Ethnic Minority Patients:	Socioeconomic disparities
	Financial strain
	Racial/ethnic disparities

(continued)

Table 17.1 (Continued)	
	Health literacy
	Barriers to navigation of health system
	Communication barriers: Cultural/language
	Fatalism
	Medical mistrust
Barriers in Older Black & Hispanic Patients:	Ageism
	SES disparities
	Health literacy
	Cultural/linguistic barriers
	Underutilization of mental health services
Protective Factors in Ethnic Minority Patients:	Spirituality
	Religion (support from religious groups)
	Kinship networks (family, friends)

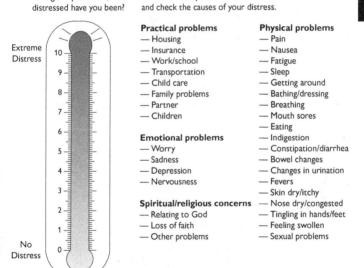

During the past week, how distressed have you been?

Please indicate your level of distress on the thermometer and check the causes of your distress.

Extreme Distress — 10

9

8

7

6

5

4

3

2

1

No Distress — 0

Practical problems
— Housing
— Insurance
— Work/school
— Transportation
— Child care
— Family problems
— Partner
— Children

Emotional problems
— Worry
— Sadness
— Depression
— Nervousness

Spiritual/religious concerns
— Relating to God
— Loss of faith
— Other problems

Physical problems
— Pain
— Nausea
— Fatigue
— Sleep
— Getting around
— Bathing/dressing
— Breathing
— Mouth sores
— Eating
— Indigestion
— Constipation/diarrhea
— Bowel changes
— Changes in urination
— Fevers
— Skin dry/itchy
— Nose dry/congested
— Tingling in hands/feet
— Feeling swollen
— Sexual problems

BRIEF SCREENING TOOL AND PROBLEM LIST

Figure 17.1 Distress Thermometer and NCCN Clinical Practice Guidelines.

Interventions to Address
Barriers to Quality Cancer Care in Older Patients of Color

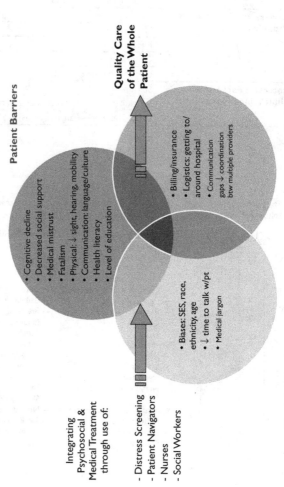

Quality Care of the Whole Patient

Patient Barriers

• Cognitive decline
• Decreased social support
• Medical mistrust
• Fatalism
• Physical: ↓ sight, hearing, mobility
• Communication: language/culture
• Health literacy
• Level of education

Healthcare Barriers

• Billing/insurance
• Logistics: getting to/ around hospital
• Communication gaps ↓ coordination btw multiple providers

Physician Barriers

• Biases: SES, race, ethnicity, age
• ↓ time to talk w/pt
• Medical jargon

Integrating Psychosocial & Medical Treatment through use of:

- Distress Screening
- Patient Navigators
- Nurses
- Social Workers

Figure 17.2 Interventions to Address Barriers to Quality Cancer Care in Older Adults of Color.

Conclusions

Despite the growing population, levels of distress, significant need for psychosocial services, and potential barriers that older minority cancer patients face, research has only recently begun to document the psychosocial issues faced by older Black and Hispanic oncology patients. In general, there has been an overall paucity of research aimed at *older Black and Hispanic cancer patients*, and as such they have "fallen through the cracks." Care must be provided for these patients in a culturally sensitive manner, taking into account language and education barriers, as well as protective factors and their impact on health-service utilization.

Below are two steps to improve the clinical care of this patient population:

1. Distress screening should be implemented, assessed and managed according to National Comprehensive Cancer Network (NCCN) clinical practice guidelines using the distress thermometer, available in English and Spanish (see Figure 17.1).[13]

2. Older Black and Hispanic patients need additional support; we have developed a preliminary theoretical model for a geriatric population that integrates psychosocial care into the medical treatment of these patients through the use of NCCN distress screening, patient navigators, nurses and social workers (see Figure 17.2).

References

1. Weiss T, Weinberger MI, Holland J, et al. Falling through the cracks: a review of psychological distress and psychosocial service needs in older Black and Hispanic patients with cancer. *Geriatr Oncol*. 2012;3(2):163–173.

2. Weiss T, Kolidas E, Stein E, et al. Psychological Distress and Psychosocial Needs Endorsed by an Underserved, Ethnically Diverse Oncology Population. Presented at the American Psychosocial Oncology Society Annual Conference, New Orleans, Louisiana, February 18–21, 2010. *Psycho-oncology* 2012;21(1):101.

3. Moadel A, Morgan C, Dutcher J. Psychosocial needs assessment among an underserved, ethnically diverse cancer patient population. *CANCER Suppl.* 2007;109:446–454.

4. Nelson CJ, Balk EM, Roth AJ. Distress, anxiety, depression, and emotional well-being in African-American men with prostate cancer. *Psycho-Oncology.* 2010; 19(10):1052–1060.

5. Meyerowitz B, Richardson J, Hudson S, et al. Ethnicity and cancer outcomes: behavioral and psychosocial considerations. *Psychological Bulletin.* 1998;123:47–70.

6. Gansler T, Henley SJ, Stein K, et al. Sociodemographic determinants of cancer treatment health literacy. *Cancer.* 2005;104:653–660.

7. Surbone A, Kagawa-Singer M, Terret C, et al. The illness trajectory of elderly cancer patients across cultures: SIOG position paper. *Ann Oncol.* 2007;18:633–638.

8. Center M, Jemal A. Cancer statistics. In: Stubblefield M, O'Dell M, eds., *Cancer Rehabilitation Principles and Practice*. New York, NY: Demos; 2009: 163.

9. Freeman HP: Poverty, culture, and social injustice: determinants of cancer disparities. *CA Cancer J Clin*. 2004;54:72–77.

10. Guidry JJ, Torrence W, Herbelin S. Closing the divide: diverse populations and cancer survivorship. *Cancer Suppl*. 2005;104(11 Suppl): 2577–2583.:

11. Ell K, Quon B, Quinn DI, et al. Improving treatment of depression among low-income patients with cancer: the design of the ADAPt-C study. *Gen Hosp Psychiat*. 2007;29:223–231.

12. Wellsi A, Zebrack B: Psychosocial barriers contributing to the under-representation of racial/ethnic minorities in cancer clinical trials. *Social Work Health Care*. 2008;46:1–14.

13. NCCN. *Distress Management, The Complete Library of NCCN Clinical Practice Guidelines in Oncology*. Jenkintown, PA, National Comprehensive Cancer Network, 2008.

Issues Specific to Common Cancer Sites

Chapter 18

Prostate Cancer

Andrew J. Roth and Mindy Greenstein

Introduction

It is estimated that about one of every six men will be diagnosed with prostate cancer during his lifetime with over 200,000 men diagnosed every year. Over 70 percent of these men are over 65 years old who will deal with a cancer diagnosis often along with other medical comorbidities, which may complicate treatment decisions. With improved diagnostics and treatment, there are more than two million survivors of prostate cancer in the United States; yet many are coping with chronic consequent physical and emotional effects or complications from their cancer treatment. Life-phase issues for these older men and their spouses or partners include retirement, relationships, and a potentially extended survivorship period with compromised quality of life from urinary, sexual, or bowel complications of treatment. About one-third of men with prostate cancer experience significant psychological distress, anxiety, or depression related to the cancer diagnosis, treatment decisions, and unpredictable complications of treatment or fear of recurrence. This distress often goes undiagnosed and untreated by their doctors.

Primary Psychosocial Issues for Older Men Regarding Prostate Cancer

- To be screened or not be screened for prostate cancer, that is the question:
  - General health and life expectancy may help in this decision.
  - Men of African descent have a higher prevalence of prostate cancer and are more often diagnosed with more advanced states of disease.
  - Men with first degree relatives already diagnosed with prostate cancer are at higher risk of getting prostate cancer themselves.
- If screened or otherwise found to have prostate cancer, should an older man (>65 years of age) have treatment or active surveillance (given that 65 percent of men with prostate cancer are over the age of 65)? Need to consider:
  - General health and life expectancy may help in this decision.
  - Genotyping for aggressiveness of tumor may also help decide which tumors need to be removed.
- If active surveillance is chosen, how to cope with uncertainty and multiple biopsies?

Table 18.1 Management of Psychosocial Issues with Prostate Cancers

Issues with Clinical Treatment	Management
Prostatectomy: Open Radical versus Laparoscopic versus Robot Assisted	
• There may be less operative bleeding, decreased pain, and shorter hospital stays and indwelling catheter placement with robot-assisted surgery. There are apparently no long-term QOL or curative differences in the surgical options.	• Experience and track record of surgeon with a particular type of surgery may be as important as the type of procedure.
• Coping with a significant risk of erectile dysfunction (ED) and potential implications for couples' intimacy or singles' (widowed, divorced, single) social lives.	• ED medication: sildenafil (Viagra®), tadalafil (Cialis®) or vardenafil (Levitra®) and penile rehabilitation. • Penile injections with vasodilating agents. • Vacutainers. • Penile suppositories. • Penile implants. • Information about realistic ranges of recovery are important to discuss with surgeons. • Couple's therapy and sex therapy can be helpful. • Cf. Chapter 7, Sexual Dysfunction.
• Coping with urinary incontinence. • Fear of urine leaking, of smelling of urine, and of having to use diapers is humiliating to many men, resulting in shunning social contact.	• Identification of etiologies and medical or surgical resolution (pelvic muscle re-education, bladder training, anticholinergic medications, artificial sphincter surgery). • Educate patients and families about incontinence. • Give recommendations to alleviate or reduce symptoms, including practicing Kegel exercises. • Encourage proper preparation with extra pads or diapers for travel. Encourage practicing allowing time for adjusting and adapting to a "new normal." Older patients can learn new tricks!
• Significant anxiety and depression.	• Counseling or medication to relieve anxiety or depressive symptoms.

(continued)

Table 18.1 (Continued)

Issues with Clinical Treatment	Management
Prostate Cancer—Radiation therapy (conventional or brachytherapy with seed implants)	
• Coping with risk of delayed erectile dysfunction and urinary problems (compared to surgery). • Coping with urinary bleeding from possible radiation cystitis.	• Support groups to gain support and perspective of other men going through similar circumstances. • Educate about protective undergarments and Kegel exercises. • Support and education from urologists and urology nurses about how to decrease urinary symptoms as well as about self-catheterization when needed is important.
• Coping with bowel function problems, such as anorectal pain, diarrhea, rectal ulceration, and bleeding.	• Support and education from gastrointestinal physicians and nursing experts to deal with bowel dysfunction is important to help these men cope with an embarrassing and socially limiting complication of treatment.
• Coping with a prostate specific antigen (PSA) level that does not fall to zero.	• Educating older men that PSA nadir may not become undetectable after radiation—as is known to happen with surgery—is important to relieve increased anxiety about uncertainty.
Prostate Cancer—Active Surveillance/Watchful waiting/Expectant Monitoring	
• No treatment side effects to deal with. • Active Surveillance is more palatable to many men to avoid QOL deficits, given the controversy over benefits of PSA Screening.	• New guidelines suggest patients discuss the benefits of screening with their physicians, rather than routine screening for all men; this is especially important for older men. Education about the significance of PSA levels is important. • Support and acknowledging fears of rising PSA levels.
• Anxiety about "doing nothing" is difficult for many men, especially those who are over age 70.	• Anxiolytic medications: Benzodiazepines such as alprazolam, 0.125 mg–0.5 mg prn; lorazepam, 0.5 mg–1 mg prn; or clonazepam, 0.25 mg–1 mg, prn may be used in the days or weeks prior to PSA testing, though caution is needed in older men.
• PSA anxiety leads to insomnia and panic symptoms.	• Antidepressants (i.e., paroxetine, sertraline, venlafaxine, citalopram, escitalopram) or buspirone for more generalized anxiety. Sedating antidepressants (e.g., mirtazapine) or atypical neuroleptics (ie, olanzapine; quetiapine) can be helpful for insomnia or for those men who cannot tolerate benzodiazepines.

(continued)

Table 18.1 (Continued)

Issues with Clinical Treatment	Management
Prostate cancer—Hormonal Treatment (Medical castration with hormones versus orchiectomy)—Gonadotropin releasing hormone (GnRH) agonists (i.e., leuprolide or goserelin) or antagonists (Degarelix) are used in conjunction with antiandrogenic agents that reduce the availability of adrenal androgens, (i.e., flutamide or bicalutamide). Abiraterone and enzalutamide are new hormonal agents. Abiraterone inhibits Cyp 17 enzymes expressed in testis, adrenals, and prostate tumor tissue, decreasing circulating levels of testosterone. Enzalutamide is an androgen receptor inhibitor. Orchiectomy is less often chosen due to body image issues, despite the greater expense of antiandrogenic medications.	
• Erectile dysfunction (ED) and decreased libido; Impact on relationships—reluctance to participate in therapy, particularly if they have never done so previously. • Concerns about bodily changes with gynecomastia or decreased testicular size; feeling emasculated. • Spouses suffer significant distress coping with their husbands' cancer.	• Education and brief psychotherapies: supportive, cognitive-behavioral, and insight-oriented for both patients and spouses/partners. • Often men are more amenable to psychotherapy if the spouse or partner is present. • Realistic goal setting. Focus on physical intimacy versus sexual performance. Sex therapy with a trained therapist can help a man express the feelings engendered by ED, and also to help a couple learn alternative ways of sharing sexual intimacy, such as with sensate focus (nongenitalia touching and massaging). Cf. Chapter 7, Sexual Dysfunction.
• Fatigue, muscular weakness and inability to conduct prior activities • Loss of usual ability to focus and diminished concentration	• Psychostimulants: methylphenidate (Ritalin®) or modafinil (Provigil®). • Activating antidepressants: fluoxetine (Prozac®) or bupropion (Wellbutrin®) improve fatigue.
• Contending with hot flashes—Symptoms are diaphoresis; drenching sweats with insomnia; feelings of intense heat, and chills. • Emotional lability, anxiety, depression and irritability • Note: Men with a history of depression may be at greater risk of becoming depressed and should be monitored for symptoms: losing interest in pleasurable and meaningful activities and social withdrawal (not primarily caused by fatigue or pain—these should be addressed), frequent passive or active thoughts about dying, constant worry about the future as a sacrifice to living a fuller life in the present.	• Antidepressants: There have been published positive results with venlafaxine (Effexor®), paroxetine (Paxil®) and sertraline (Zoloft®) and gabapentin (Neurontin®) improving hot flashes. • Pulse the hormonal therapy intermittently in 6–12 month intervals. • Decrease caffeine, alcohol, and hot fluid intake. • Psychotropic medications can be effective for changes in mood and anxiety. Start low doses and go slowly (cf. Chapter 4).

(continued)

Table 18.1 (Continued)

Issues with Clinical Treatment	Management
Prostate cancer—Chemotherapy and Advanced Disease	
• Anxiety/fear, fatigue, nausea, pain.	• Cf. Chapter 6, Anxiety Disorders, and Chapter 7, Anxiety/fear: Consider supportive therapy and relaxation exercises for anxiety and fear and/or lorazepam during chemotherapy—it will also help nausea. Monitor for cognitive and coordination deficits in the elderly. Fatigue: Consider behavioral activation, psychostimulants for fatigue and cognitive reframing. • Prostate cancer may metastasize to bones, which can be painful. Older men are often reluctant to take pain medications or dosages adequate to truly help, fearing side effects or feeling embarrassed that they cannot handle the pain. It is important to encourage treatment of pain from metastasis and manage the side effects of pain medication to make the risk vs. benefit ratio of taking pain medications far in favor of pain relief. Cf. Chapter 7, Pain. • Cf. Chapter 7, Pain.
• End of life issues: "I used to be such a strong guy, and look at me now... what good am I?" "I'm gonna die; why continue living like this... I should die now."	• Help the patient find activities appropriate to his energy level and performance status. • Modeling for adult children, grandchildren, spouses/partners and friends how to face one of the greatest challenges to humans with appropriate emotional reactions, humor, acceptance of the things we cannot change but a desire to appreciate and enjoy the things still under our control (rather than a superhero's grin and bear it or stoical response), can be one of the most important legacies of wisdom a man (or anyone) may pass down to others.

- If active treatment is selected, which treatment will give the best longevity and least risk to quality of life (QOL) among various options for surgery and/or radiation therapy?
- After treatment, how can older men best cope with:
  - Multiple late-life health and social concerns and changes.
  - Male body and sexual image and changes in functioning due to treatment.
  - Fatigue.

See Table 18.1.

Summary

The most prominent psychosocial issues in older men with prostate cancer are decisions about treatment options, including active surveillance or no treatment. Coping with changes in sexuality, bladder and bowel function, body image, relationships, and lifestyle are challenges facing these older men and their spouses or partners. In advanced prostate cancer, libido as well as erectile functioning is primarily affected by hormonal treatments that cause androgen ablation. The tumor marker PSA that is used to follow treatment outcomes often creates significant anxiety. New treatments for advanced prostate cancer are giving new hope to patients, who feel they have more realistic hope of living long enough to be able to take advantage of the next new treatment that will arrive. Urinary incontinence is usually a common, transient problem with surgical or radiation therapy for prostate cancer, yet it may become a longer-term challenge that can be adjusted to. Patients with advanced prostate cancer may have to deal with the pain of bone metastases, and may need to be encouraged to take medication to relieve their pain. Psychologically, they and their spouses/partners may benefit from counseling to help cope with the knowledge of poor prognosis and mortality.

Management of these problems is best done by means of:

- Education and support about illness and treatment.
- Individual and group psychotherapy.
- Couples and/or sex therapy.
- Referral to a specialist for erectile dysfunction.
- Behavioral and Relaxation interventions.
- Psychotropic medications for symptoms of distress, fatigue, or hot flashes.

References

1. Alsadius D, Olsson C, Pettersson N, Tucker SL, Wilderäng U, Steineck G. Perception of body odor—an overlooked consequence of long-term gastro-intestinal and urinary symptoms after radiation therapy for prostate cancer. J Cancer Surviv. 2013;7(4):652–658.

2. Bergman J, Litwin MS. Quality of life in men undergoing active surveillance for localized prostate cancer. J Natl Cancer Inst Monogr. 2012;(45):242–249.

3. Chambers SK, Zajdlewicz L, Youlden DR, Holland JC, Dunn J. The valid-ity of the distress thermometer in prostate cancer populations. Psychooncol. 2014;23:195–203.

4. Cherrier MM, Anderson K, David D, et al. A randomized trial of cognitive rehabilitation in cancer survivors. Life Sci. 2013;93(17):617–622.

5. Chipperfield K, Fletcher J, Millar J, et al. Predictors of depression, anxiety and quality of life in patients with prostate cancer receiving androgen depri-vation therapy. Psychooncol. Mar 2013;22(10):2169–2176.

6. Kornblith AB, Herr HW, Ofman US, Scher HI & Holland JC. Quality of life of patients with prostate cancer and their spouses. The value of a database in clinical care. Cancer. 1994;73:2791–2802.

7. Nelson CJ, Gilley J, Roth AJ. The impact of a cancer diagnosis on sexual health. In: *Cancer and Sexual Health*, Mulhall JP, ed. New York, NY: Human Press; 2011.

8. Nelson CJ, Kenowitz J. Communication and intimacy-enhancing interventions for men diagnosed with prostate cancer and their partners. *J Sex Med*. 2013;(Suppl 10)1:127–132.

9. Roth A, Nelson CJ, Rosenfeld B, et al. Assessing anxiety in men with prostate cancer: further data on the reliability and validity of the Memorial Anxiety Scale for Prostate Cancer (MAX-PC). *Psychosomatics*. 2006;47(4):340–347.

10. Zaider T, Manne S, Nelson C, Mulhall J, Kissane D. Loss of masculine identity, marital affection, and sexual bother in men with localized prostate cancer. *J Sex Med*. 2012;9(10):2724–2732.

Chapter 19

Psychosocial Issues Specific to Breast Cancer

Matthew N. Doolittle and Mary Jane Massie

Breast Cancer

Breast cancer is the most common cancer in women and is second only to lung cancer in cancer deaths in women. Over 232,000 women in the United States are diagnosed with invasive breast cancer yearly, and about 40,000 women will die. Forty-one percent of breast cancer diagnoses occur in women over the age of 65. Although more than 85% of women diagnosed with Stage I breast cancer will be alive in 5 years, survival drops dramatically when cancers are diagnosed at later stages. A woman's ability to manage a breast cancer diagnosis and treatment commonly changes over the course of illness and depends on medical, psychological and social factors.[1]

Evaluation

The severity of the cancer itself, psychiatric history and prior level of functioning, level of social and emotional supports, and stage of life all affect patients' adjustment to cancer diagnosis and treatment (Table 19.1). Many women adapt well to the diagnosis and treatment of cancer with the support of family, oncologists, nurses, social workers, and clergy, and do not require psychiatric support. A subset of women should be referred for psychiatric consultation (Table 19.2). Older women may be reluctant to seek psychiatry, and may benefit from education about how frequently cancer patients experience psychological distress, and about the support that can be provided by psychiatry. In the case of some elderly patients, decreased reserve, decreased social supports, clinical bias toward undertreatment, and a particular sensitivity to effective medical communication may cause psychosocial burdens particular to this age group (Table 19.3). Some areas including sexual function that may receive less attention in the elderly may nonetheless affect quality of life just a significantly for many older patients (Table 19.4). Although in general older patients are more likely to be referred for surgery for cancer treatment, the decision to undergo prophylactic mastectomy or oophorectomy can be more complicated in older age groups, and consideration of psychiatric risks of older women contemplating surgery is at least as important as it is in the case of younger women

Table 19.1 Factors Affecting Adjustment to Diagnosis and Treatment[2,3]

- The disease itself (stage at diagnosis, type of treatments recommended, symptoms, clinical course, and prognosis)
- Prior level of adjustment, patient's own personality and coping style and prior experience with loss
- The threat that breast cancer poses to attaining age-appropriate development goals (e.g., career, retirement)
- Cultural, spiritual and religious attitudes
- Prior depression or anxiety
- Cognitive function
- Presence of emotionally supportive persons
- Potential for physical and psychological rehabilitation

Table 19.2 Reasons for Psychiatric Consult

Psychiatric Consult Indicated Current Symptoms/History of:	Consider Psychiatric Consult Facing Difficult Decisions:
• Depression and anxiety	• How to deal with family history of breast cancer
• Suicidal thinking or attempt (urgent consult)	• Whether to undergo genetic testing
• Alcohol or other abuse	• Whether to inform family of results of genetic testing
• Confusional state, delirium, or encephalopathy (urgent consult)	• Whether to have risk-reducing surgery such as prophylactic mastectomy and/or prophylactic oophorectomy after a cancer diagnosis or if BRCA 1 or 2 mutation carrier
• Mood swings, insomnia, or irritability from steroids	• Whether to have contralateral prophylactic mastectomy, as risk-reducing surgery
• Questions about capacity to consent to treatment	• Whether to have mastectomy or limited resection followed by irradiation
• Very old or alone	• Whether to have breast reconstruction following mastectomy
• Adjusting to multiple losses	• If having reconstruction, which natural tissue or implant to select
• Managing multiple life stresses	• Whether or when to tell employer, colleagues, friends, new relationship/sexual partner about current breast cancer treatment or cancer history
• Paralyzed by cancer-treatment decisions	
• Fear death during surgery or terrified by loss of control under anesthesia	
• Request euthanasia	

41% of breast cancer occurs in women over age 65; older women may be less likely than younger women to seek psychiatric consultation.

Table 19.3 Issues Especially Relevant to Older Breast Cancer Patients

- **Psychiatric Risk**. Though literature has focused on the needs of younger women who are disproportionately represented among those seeking psychiatric help after cancer diagnosis, rates of depression after breast cancer diagnosis are similar among younger and older women, and though the elderly seem more resilient in some ways, overall quality of life after cancer diagnosis may be worse among the elderly than among the young.[4,5]

- **Decreased Functional and Cognitive Reserve**. A breast cancer diagnosis is evidence of further decline of health in women who may already be facing various health issues as well as medical and social losses (poor vision, hearing problems, other chronic or life-threatening conditions, bereavement, life disappointments, etc.) General health and well-being decline in elderly patients after breast cancer diagnosis.

- **Decreased Social Support**. Many elderly patients are alone and geographically separated from family, and even those who are not alone may have partners with chronic illnesses that limit their ability to provide support even as patients face greater logistical and emotional needs.

- **Undertreatment**. Though more likely to be offered mastectomy, older patients are less likely to be offered chemotherapy than younger patients, and Medicare policies complicate access to some treatments.[6]

- **Physical and Functional Disability**. Older patients are more likely than younger patients to have ongoing physical limitations after breast cancer treatment, and they may be especially vulnerable to psychological distress associated with these limitations.

- **Body Image**. Though literature has focused on younger patients, altered body image is a significant cause of psychological distress in elderly patients undergoing breast cancer surgery.[4]

- **Medical Communications**. The quality of medical interactions seems especially important in causing or relieving distress in elderly patients.[7]

- **Mammography**: Elderly women are less likely to undergo breast cancer screening than younger women and public health and education campaigns do focus on regular mammograms. Major cancer organizations advocate screening until age 70–75. However, follow-up mammography may not be recommended for older women with previously diagnosed breast cancer if any findings would not alter treatment decisions. This apparent departure may make older women feel unsafe, or even abandoned or hopeless.

The hereditary breast cancer syndrome accounts for only 5–7% of all breast cancer cases. Some elderly women will inquire about testing for BRCA1 and 2. In addition, depending on risk factors, older women may elect to undergo prophylactic mastectomy or oophorectomy, although these procedures are less common in the elderly than in younger patients.

Table 19.4 Major Sexual Issues in Postmenopausal Breast Cancer Patients

- Decreased libido (desire)
- Decreased vaginal lubrication
- Painful sex
- Decreased pleasure in sex
- Embarrassment about drains, scars, implants, alopecia, lymphedema, weight gain or loss

Table 19.5 Components of the Psychiatric Evaluation of Women Who Consider Prophylactic Mastectomy and/or Prophylactic Oophorectomy

- Family cancer history
- Personal history of breast, ovarian cancer, and other cancers
- Psychiatric history
- Anxiety disorder
- Depressive disorder
- Body dysmorphic disorder
- Personality disorder
- Perception of cancer risk and anxiety associated with perceptions
- Understanding of actual risk
- Satisfaction with previous plastic surgeries
- Litigation history
- History of abuse, rape, or assault
- Sexual, pregnancy, and breast-feeding history
- Many older women are responsible for the care of young relatives or elderly partners, and these obligations may affect decisions
- Partner's role in the consideration of prophylactic surgery
- Availability of strategies to reduce anxiety, regardless of the patient's decision

Table 19.6 Burdens of the Patient's Partner/Husband/Children[8,9]

- Facing uncertainty, fear of death, and loss of control
- Participating in many doctor appointments and everyday care
- Continuing work; managing diminished finances
- Managing additional responsibility, such as domestic responsibilities
- Adjusting to altered appearance and temporary (or permanent) loss of sexual partner
- Caring for a partner who may at times seem ungrateful, irritable, depressed

(Table 19.5). Similarly, although the burden faced by partners and families of elderly patients may be different from that faced by the families of patients in an earlier stage of life characterized by different responsibilities, the challenge can be equally significant in the older population (Table 19.6).

Interventions

Psychosocial interventions for women with breast cancer include medications, individual and group psychotherapy, specialized programs, and complementary treatments. In addition to following dosing guidelines for the elderly, particular caution should be used when prescribing hypnotics and benzodiazepines to elderly patients (Table 19.7). Psychiatric side effects of antiandrogens used in cancer treatment can be burdensome, and although in the elderly population tamoxifen is less likely to be prescribed than aromatase inhibitors, awareness of both general recommendations and the contra-indications in patients using tamoxifen is important for the psycho-oncologist

Table 19.7 Pharmacological Interventions for Breast Cancer Patients*

General Considerations	• Psychoactive medications should be dosed with care in the elderly; initial target doses might be half those typical for younger people, with increases if necessary and well-tolerated.
Presurgery, pre- and postchemotherapy, anxiety/agitation	• Polypharmacy is a risk especially in the elderly
	• Medication review and reconciliation is recommended at every visit
Nausea pre- and postchemotherapy	• Benzodiazepines, hypnotics, and anticholinergics should be used with caution owing to risk of falls, cognitive side effects, and increased risk of delirium
Insomnia	
Depression, panic, generalized anxiety	• Neuroleptics may have cardiovascular risks especially in patients with cognitive impairment, but benefits of temporary treatment for agitation, delirium, or nausea may outweigh risks
Vasomotor menopausal symptoms (hot flashes)	• Anxiolytics—lorazepam (Ativan®), alprazolam (Xanax®), clonazepam (Klonopin®), see caution earlier
Unrelenting fatigue after chemotherapy or irradiation	• Neuroleptics—haloperidol (Haldol®), olanzapine (Zyprexa®), see caution earlier
Postmastectomy neuropathic pain; peripheral neuropathy	• Anxiolytics—lorazepam (Ativan®), alprazolam (Xanax®), clonazepam (Klonopin®), see caution earlier
	• Antiemetics—ondansetron (Zofran®), anticholinergic antiemetics with caution
	• Antidepressants—mirtazapine (Remeron®), trazodone (Oleptro®)
	• Hypnotics are not first-line agents in the elderly, may be used with caution; maximum dose is half that for younger people—zolpidem (Ambien®), eszopiclone (Lunesta®)
	• Benzodiazepines are not first-line agents in the elderly, may be used with caution—lorazepam (Ativan®), temazepam (Restoril®)
	• Antidepressants—sertraline (Zoloft®), paroxetine (Paxil®), duloxetine (Cymbalta®), escitalopram (Lexapro®), fluoxetine (Prozac®), citalopram (Celexa®)*
	• Antidepressants—sertraline (Zoloft®), paroxetine (Paxil®), venlafaxine (Effexor®)*
	• Psychostimulants—modafinil (Provigil®), methylphenidate (Ritalin®)
	• Antidepressants—duloxetine (Cymbalta®)
	• Anticonvulsants—gabapentin (Neurontin®)
	• Tricyclic antidepressants—nortriptyline (Pamelor®), amitriptyline (Elavil®), not first-line agents in the elderly
	• Analgesics

*Recommended with tamoxifen: venlafaxine, mirtazapine.

(Table 19.9). Nonpharmacological interventions including individual therapy, group therapy, and community-based programs can be just as important as medications in improving the quality of life of elderly patients (Table 19.8). Metastatic breast cancer poses particular challenges, and group and individual psychiatric interventions can play an important role in helping these patients address practical and existential concerns (Table 19.10). Although increasing attention has been paid to younger populations with breast cancer, it remains true that a substantial percentage of breast cancers occur in women over the age of 65. Psychosocial issues in this population are in some respects similar to those in younger populations, even in some areas thought to be more relevant to younger patients. In addition, older patients have particular areas of vulnerability less relevant to younger groups. Consideration of psychosocial burdens is important for good care in the elderly breast cancer patient, from evaluating psychiatric risk at the time of diagnosis, assisting in treatment decisions, managing side effects, and addressing concerns about the end of life.

Table 19.8 Nonpharmacological Interventions for Breast Cancer Patients[10]

Psychotherapy

Patients at all stages; those who need to make treatment decisions

Patients at time of diagnosis, with relapse or with metastatic disease

Specialized Programs

Appearance during chemotherapy

Sexual dysfunction

Lymphedema

Nutrition and avoiding weight gain

Fitting for appropriate prosthesis

Complementary Treatments

Hot flashes

Chemotherapy or irradiation

- Individual Therapy—supportive, exploratory, psychodynamic, cognitive and behavioral elements
- Group Therapy—supportive, cognitive, and behavioral elements
- Look Good…Feel Better® (www.lookgoodfeelbetter.org)
- Sexual counseling, rehabilitation
- Physical therapy
- Nutritional counseling
- Prosthetic consultants
- Acupuncture
- Gentle exercise and toning—Yoga, Pilates, Tai Chi

Table 19.9 Interventions for Psychiatric Side Effects of Antiestrogens

Symptom	Intervention
Irritability	• Antidepressants—sertraline (Zoloft®), paroxetine (Paxil®), escitalopram (Lexapro®), fluoxetine (Prozac®), citalopram (Celexa®), see below if tamoxifen • Anxiolytics—lorazepam (Ativan®), alprazolam (Xanax®), clonazepam (Klonopin®), see caution in Table 19.7
Depression	• Antidepressants
Insomnia	• Antidepressants—mirtazapine (Remeron®), trazodone (Oleptro®) • Caution with hypnotics, benzodiazepines in the elderly, see Table 19.7
Hot-flashes/ night-sweats	• Serotonin norepinephrine reuptake inhibitors (SNRI's)— venlafaxine (Effexor®) • Selective serotonin reuptake inhibitors (SSRI's)—sertraline (Zoloft®), paroxetine (Paxil®), see below if tamoxifen
Weight gain	• Nutrition consult
Use with tamoxifen	• Paroxetine (Paxil®), fluoxetine (Prozac®), bupropion (Wellbutrin®)
Avoid with tamoxifen	• Paroxetine (Paxil®), fluoxetine (Prozac®), bupropion (Wellbutrin®)

Women who are eligible for antiestrogen therapy (tamoxifen, raloxifene, anastrazole, and exemestane) are treated for years.

Table 19.10 Benefits of Individual or Group Psychiatric Intervention in Addressing Major Issues with Metastatic Breast Cancer

Issues	Benefits
• Adjusting to pain and fear of pain, as well as physical and cognitive deterioration • Mourning the loss of autonomous function, former roles, hopes, and aspirations • Altering, reducing and/or phasing out work or other commitments • Managing life disruption due to many outpatient visits and hospitalizations • Living with health uncertainty that may complicate everyday and long-term planning • Preparing children and other loved ones both emotionally and practically for death • Adapting to a series of treatments, knowing that treatment is offered without hope for cure • Considering practical issues about where to die, funeral or memorial services, bequests, etc. • Living with fear of death	• Opportunity to address existential, physical, emotional, social, psychosexual concerns, and issues in relationships with family and others • Opportunity to express emotions, gain support, manage anxiety, fear, depression • Source of meaningful information • Challenge pessimistic thoughts • Consider priorities • Manage treatment side effects (promote adherence to cancer treatment) • Phase specific issues (i.e., preparation for death)

References

1. Howlader N, Noone AM, Krapcho M, et al., eds. *SEER Cancer Statistics Review, 1975–2010*, Bethesda, MD: National Cancer Institute. http://seer.cancer.gov/csr/1975_2010/ based on November 2012 SEER data submission, posted to the SEER website, April 2013.

2. Jim HSL, Small BJ, Minton S, Andrykowski M, Jacobsen PB. History of major depressive disorder prospectively predicts a worse quality of life in women with breast cancer. *Ann Behav Med.* 2012;43:402–408.

3. Lim CC, Devi MK, Ang E. Anxiety in women with breast cancer undergoing treatment: a systemic review. *Int J Evid Based Healthc.* 2011;9:215–235.

4. Kornblith, A. B., Powell, M., Regan, M. M., et al. Long-term psychosocial adjustment of older vs younger survivors of breast and endometrial cancer. *Psychooncology.* 2007;16(10): 895–903. doi:10.1002/pon.1146 [doi]

5. Park, B. W., Lee, S., Lee, A. R., Lee, K. H., Hwang, S. Y. Quality of life differences between younger and older breast cancer patients. *J. Breast Cancer.* 2011;14(2):112–118.

6. Swaby, R. F., & Goldstein, L. J. A prospective, longitudinal study of the functional status and quality of life of older patients with breast cancer receiving adjuvant chemotherapy. *Breast Diseases.* 2007;18(3), 312–313.

7. Clough-Gorr, K. M., Ganz, P. A., Silliman, R. A. Older breast cancer survivors: Factors associated with change in emotional well-being. *J Clin Oncol,* 2007;25(11):1334–1340. doi:JCO.2006.09.8665 [pii] 10.1200/JCO.2006.09.8665 [doi]

8. Kroenke CH, Quesenberry C, Kwan ML et al. Social networks, social support, and burden in relationships, and mortality after breast cancer diagnosis in the Life After Breast Cancer Epidemiology (LACE) study. *Breast Cancer Res Treat.* 2013;137:261–271.

9. Northouse L, Williams AL, Given B, McCorkle R. Psychosocial care for family caregivers of patients with cancer. *J Clin Oncol.* 2012;30:1227–1234.

10. Alfano CM, Ganz PA, Rowland JH, Hahn EE. Cancer survivorship and cancer rehabilitation: revitalizing the link. *J Clin Oncol.* 2012;30:904–906.

Chapter 20

Lung Cancer

R. Garrett Key

Geriatric patients account for approximately 65 percent of all lung cancer cases[1] and the fastest growing group of lung cancer patient is over 80 years of age.[2] The relatively poor prognosis for lung cancer patients and high frequency with which their disease is discovered at advanced stage underscore the need to address concerns about death and dying. This is even more pertinent in the elderly as survival decreases with age at diagnosis. Geriatric lung patients, particularly the fit elderly, likely get similar benefit from standard treatments as patients younger patients but are not treated with the modalities as often with advancing age. This is reflected in a reduced relative survival rate for older patients. See Tables 20.1 and 20.2.

Lung cancer patients have an increased burden of physical symptoms when compared to other cancers and increased rates of psychological distress. Common causes of distress in cancer patients are fatigue, pain, depression, insomnia, anxiety, and dyspnea. In the geriatric population, social functioning and physical symptom burden predict depression.[4] Surgically cured patients continue to have increased rates of depression and anxiety following treatment and should be assessed in follow-up visits. Notably, association between disease stage or treatment type and the level of distress has not been found.[5]

Table 20.1 5-Year Survival Rates for NSCLC by Stage at Diagnosis, 2001–2007[3]		
Localized disease	**Regional Spread**	**Distant Metastasis**
52%	24%	4%
American Cancer Society. *Cancer Facts & Figures 2012*. Atlanta, GA: Author; 2012.		

Table 20.2 5-Year Relative Survival Rates by Age Group		
Age <70 years	**Age 70–79 years**	**Age**
15.5%	12.3%	7.4%
Owonikoko TK, Ragin CC, Belani CP, et al. Lung cancer in elderly patients: an analysis of the surveillance, epidemiology, and end results database. *J Clin Oncol*. 2007;25(35):5570–5577.		

Fears about unmitigated physical suffering, breathlessness, and brain metastasis are common concerns, and patients will benefit from education about the tools for symptom control that exist. Early introduction of palliative care for patients with metastatic disease has been found to improve quality of life, decrease rates of depression, reduce aggressive end-of-life care, and lengthen survival.[6]

Patients with more complex, severe, or refractory symptoms should be referred to a mental health specialist, preferably with experience working in the context of cancer or chronic illness. See Table 20.3.

Fatigue

Moderate to severe fatigue is found in 40 percent of lung cancer patients at the time of initial presentation and may increase to 90 percent through the course of treatment.[8] Patients should be screened regularly for fatigue, educated on cancer related fatigue, and encouraged to use energy conservation strategies. See Box 20.1 and Table 20.4.

Table 20.3 Most Limiting Symptoms in Geriatric Lung Cancer Patients[7]

Symptom	Frequency
Fatigue	79%
Dyspnea	58%
Weakness	57%
Vomiting	15%
Incoordination	16%
Pain	60%
Insomnia	49%
Nausea	34%
Poor concentration	16%

Adapted from Gift AG, Jablonski A, Stommel M, Given CW. Symptom clusters in elderly patients with lung cancer. *Oncol Nurs Forum*. 2004;31(2):202–212.

Box 20.1 Treatable Comorbidities Contributing to Fatigue

- Anemia.
- Sleep disturbance.
- Pain.
- Electrolyte imbalance.
- Nutritional deficiency.
- Inactivity/Deconditioning.

Table 20.4 Treatment of Cancer Related Fatigue

Treatment	Notes
Exercise (30–60 mins daily walking)	Strongest evidence for efficacy Physical therapy referral for weakness or cachexia
Methylphenidate (Ritalin®) 5–20 mg BID PRN	May be used PRN Caution in cardiac disease May also benefit cognition/wakefulness
Modafinil (Provigil®) 50–200 mg daily Armodafinil (NuVigil®) 50–250 mg daily	Caution with cardiac disease Reduce dosage in severe hepatic impairment May also benefit cognition/wakefulness

Box 20.2 Physiological Causes of Dyspnea

- Pulmonary Embolus.
- Pneumonia.
- COPD/Asthma.
- Sepsis.
- Anemia.
- Parenchymal metastasis.
- Lymphangitic carcinomatosis.
- Airway obstruction by tumor.
- Ascites.
- Respiratory muscle weakness.

Table 20.5 Pharmacotherapy for Breathlessness/Dyspnea

Treatment	Notes
Opioids	Proven benefit for subjective air hunger Caution for respiratory depression and synergy with other CNS depressants
Supplemental Oxygen	Mixed evidence for patients without hypoxemia
Corticosteroids	Limited evidence for efficacy
Benzodiazepines	NOT effective for physiologically based anxiety

Anxiety and Dyspnea

Problematic anxiety may be found in 25 percent or more of lung cancer patients.[9] Treatment of anxiety in lung cancer requires separation of physiologically based symptoms from psychologically based anxiety. See Box 20.2 and Tables 20.5–20.7.

Table 20.6 Nonpharmacological Palliative Treatment of Dyspnea/Breathlessness

Strength of Evidence	Intervention
High	Neuromuscular electrical stimulation of breathing muscles
	Chest wall vibration
Moderate	Walking aids
	Breathing training
Low	Acupuncture/acupressure
No evidence for efficacy	Music therapy
Insufficient data	Relaxation therapy
	Counseling and support
	Case management
	Psychotherapy

Adapted from Bausewein C BS, Gysels M, Higginson I. Non-pharmacological interventions for breathlessness in advanced stages of malignant and non-malignant disease. *Cochrane Database Syst Rev.* 2008(2).

Table 20.7 Pharmacotherapy of Nonphysiologic Anxiety

SSRI: Citalopram (Celexa®) 10–20 mg daily Escitalopram (Lexapro®) 5–10 mg daily	Minimal drug interactions, no 2D6 inhibition Helpful for comorbid depression
SNRI: Venlafaxine ER (Effexor XR®) 37.5–225 mg daily	May offer benefit to neuropathic pain Beneficial for comorbid depression
Benzodiazepines: Intermittent use: • Lorazepam(Ativan®) 0.5–2 mg BID/TID PRN Chronic anxiety: • Clonazepam (Klonopin®) 0.25–2 mg BID • Alprazolam (Xanax®) 0.125–2 mg BID/TID	Rapid efficacy Short term benefit for insomnia Caution for sedation in elderly Caution in conjunction with opioids/CNS depressants May worsen cognition, increase fall risk Minimal dose and duration of treatment preferred
Alpha 2 antagonist: Mirtazapine (Remeron®) 7.5–45 mg QHS	Beneficial for insomnia Improves nausea/appetite Caution for SIADH, orthostasis, anticholinergic side effects Elderly may have decreased clearance
Buspirone (BuSpar®) 7.5–30 mg BID	Decreased clearance in renal/hepatic impairment
Atypical Antipsychotic: Olanzapine (Zyprexa®) 2.5–10 mg QHS	Collateral benefit for appetite/nausea/insomnia More rapid onset of action than SSRI Black box warning for increased risk of death in elderly with dementia-related psychosis

Insomnia

Insomnia is common in lung cancer and pain, nausea, dyspnea, anxiety, and depressed mood may be contributing factors. Geriatric patients may be more sensitive to sedating- or delirium-inducing effects of hypnotics; thus, they should be used judiciously. Nonpharmacologic treatments should be attempted first. Persistent sleep problems warrant referral to a sleep specialist. See Tables 20.8 and 20.9.

Table 20.8 Basic Nonpharmacologic Interventions for Insomnia

Treatment	Notes
Stimulus Control	Only use bed for sleep
	Only attempt to sleep when tired
	Leave bed if unable to sleep
	Maintain regular waking time
	Limit napping to <30 mins daily
Sleep Hygiene Education	Regular daytime exercise, not at night
	No tobacco, caffeine, alcohol, stimulants near bedtime
	Minimize heavy food/drink near bedtime
	Avoid naps late in day
	Maintain regular bedtime/wake time routine
	Avoid stimulating activity near bedtime
	Avoid clock watching in bed
Sleep Restriction	Use a sleep log to calculate total time sleeping nightly
	Only remain in bed for total time spent sleeping
	Maintain set wake time and adjust bedtime accordingly
Relaxation Therapies	Progressive muscle relaxation techniques
	Meditation focused on psychological arousal

Adapted from Krishnan P, Hawranik P. Diagnosis and management of geriatric insomnia: a guide for nurse practitioners. *J Am Acad Nurse Practition*. 2008;20(12):590–599.

Table 20.9 Pharmacotherapy for Insomnia

Medication	Notes
Melatonin 3–5 mg given 3–4 h before sleep	Evidence for efficacy is lacking
	Supplement content not FDA regulated
Ramelteon (Rozerem®) 8mg QHS	Melatonin receptor agonist
	Caution with hepatic/renal impairment
Trazodone (Desyrel®) 25–100 mg QHS	Serotonin reuptake inhibitor
	Sleep dose lower than typical effective antidepressant dose

Table 20.9 (Continued)

Eszopiclone (Lunesta®) 1–2 mg QHS	Only medication approved for long term use
Zaleplon (Sonata®) 5 mg QHS or PRN early waking	May be taken for waking during night
Mirtazapine (Remeron®) 7.5–15 mg QHS	May also benefit nausea/appetite
	Antidepressant benefit may require higher dosage
	Caution for SIADH, orthostasis, anticholinergic side effects
	Elderly may have decreased clearance

Box 20.3 Indicators of Depression in Cancer Patients

• Tearfulness, depressed appearance.
• Social withdrawal, decreased talkativeness.
• Brooding, self-pity, pessimism.
• Lack of reactivity.

Endicott J. Measurement of depression in patients with cancer. *Cancer.* 1984;53(Suppl 10): 2243–2249.

Depression

Depression is common in lung cancer, found in up to one third of patients at diagnosis. The most significant risk factor for depression in lung cancer is functional impairment.[12] Hypoactive delirium may mimic depression and should be ruled out. See Box 20.3.

No RCTs specific to treatment of depression in lung cancer patients exist.[14] Typical treatment strategies are employed in conjunction with early, aggressive palliation of physical symptoms. See Table 20.10.

Tobacco Cessation

Smoking cessation should be aggressively pursued for all smokers. Smoking accounts for 30 percent of all cancer deaths and 80 percent of lung cancer deaths. Light or "low tar" cigarette use does not reduce the risk of lung cancer. There is evidence that smoking cessation can offer more than twofold improvement in long-term survival for early stage lung cancer.[15] The benefits of smoking cessation in advanced cancer are less clear, but increased time to progression and prolonged survival are suggested. See Box 20.4 and Tables 20.11 and 20.12.

Table 20.10 Pharmacotherapy of Depression in Lung Cancer

Class	Notes
SSRI: Citalopram (Celexa®) 10–20 mg daily	Minimal drug interactions, no 2D6 inhibition
Escitalopram (Lexapro®) 5–10 mg daily	Helpful for comorbid anxiety
SNRI: Venlafaxine ER (Effexor XR®) 37.5–225 mg daily	May offer benefit to neuropathic pain
	May be more helpful for more anergic depression
NDRI: Bupropion ER (Wellbutrin XL®) 100–450 mg daily	Effective for smoking cessation
	Effective for inattention
	May exacerbate anxiety/insomnia
Alpha 2 antagonist: Mirtazapine (Remeron®) 7.5–45 mg QHS	Beneficial for insomnia
	Improves nausea/appetite
	Caution for SIADH, orthostasis, anticholinergic side effects
	Elderly may have decreased clearance

Box 20.4 Brief Cessation Counseling Strategies

ASK about tobacco use.
ADVISE cessation.
ASSESS readiness to quit.
ASSIST with education and pharmacotherapy.
ARRANGE for follow up.

Agency for Healthcare Research and Quality. *Treating Tobacco Use and Dependence.* Rockville, MD: Author; 2013. http://www.ahrq.gov/professionals/clinicians-providers/guidelines-recommendations/tobacco/clinicians/update/index.html

Neurologically Manifested Paraneoplastic Syndromes

Paraneoplastic syndromes are common in lung cancer patients, and those with neuropsychiatric manifestations have been estimated as high as 5 percent.[17] They are most common in small cell lung cancer patients, are not always reversible, and typically portend a poor prognosis. See Table 20.13.

Table 20.11 Smoking Cessation Pharmacotherapy Guidelines

Pharmacotherapy	Dosage	Duration	Precautions/Contraindications	Adverse Effects	Patient Education

• Nicotine Patch
NicoDerm CQ®
Habitrol®
	If smoking 11 cig/d or >:
	• 21 mg/24 hr
	• 14 mg/24 hr
	• 7 mg/24 hr
	If smoking 10 cig/d or <:
	• 14 mg/24 hr
	• 7 mg/24 hr
		• 6 weeks
		• 2 weeks
		• 2 weeks
		• 6 weeks
		• 2 weeks
			• Uncontrolled Hypertension	• Skin irritation
				  Redness
				  Swelling
				  itching
				• Disruption in
				  Sleep
				  Nightmares
				  Vivid dreams
					• Instruct patient to rotate patch site daily
					• Instruct patient to remove patch prior to bedtime if sleep is disrupted and bothersome.

• Nicotine Polacrilex Gum **Nicorette Gum**®	• **2 mg** if smoking 24 or < cig/d • **4 mg** if smoking 25 or > cig/d • Do not exceed 24 pieces of gum/24 hr	• Up to 12 weeks	• Poor dentition • Xerostomia	• Hiccups • Upset stomach • Jaw ache	• Chew gum on a fixed schedule • "Chew & Park" each piece of gum for 30 minutes • Avoid eating/drinking anything except water 15 minutes before & during chewing
• Nicotine Lozenge **Commit**®	• **2 mg** if smoking the first cigarette **more than** 30 minutes after waking up • **4 mg** if smoking the first cigarette **within** 30 minutes after waking up	• Up to 12 weeks	• Xerostomia	• Local irritation to mouth & throat • Upset stomach	• Avoid eating/drinking anything except water 15 minutes before & during when using a lozenge • Each lozenge will take 20–30 minutes to dissolve

Medication	Dosage	Duration	Contraindications	Side Effects	Instructions
	• Do not use more than 20 lozenges/ 24 hr				
Nicotine Inhalation System **Nicotrol Inhaler**®	• 6–16 cartridges/day	• Up to 6 months		• Local irritation to mouth & throat • Upset stomach	• Each cartridge will take 80–100 inhalations over 20 minutes • Instruct patient to puff on inhalers like a cigar. Absorption is in the buccal mucosa.
Bupropion **Zyban**® **Wellbutrin SR**®	• 150 mg daily x 3 days **THEN** • 150 mg BID	• 12 weeks	• History of seizures • History of eating disorders Bulimia Anorexia	• Insomnia • Dry mouth • Restlessness • Dizziness	• Overlap with smoking for 1–2 weeks • Does not need to be tapered off
Varenicline **Chantix**®	• Days 1–3: 0.5 mg daily THEN • Days 4–7: 0.5 mg BID THEN • Days 8–End of treatment: 1 mg BID	• 12 weeks • If the patient has quit smoking, may be given another 12 weeks of treatment to prevent relapse.	• Kidney problems or undergoing dialysis • Pregnant or planning on getting pregnant • Breast feeding	• Mild nausea • Sleep problems • Headaches	• Take medication with a full glass of water after you eat a meal. • Allow 8 hours between each dose • Take this medication a few hours before bedtime to avoid restlessness

Table 20.12 Contacts for Tobacco Cessation Programs

• National Cancer Institute (NCI)	www.smokefree.gov	1-877-448-7848
• American Cancer Society	www.cancer.org	1-800-ACS-2345
• American Lung Association	www.lungusa.org	1-800-LUNG-USA
• American Heart Association	www.americanheart.org	1-800-242-8721
• U.S.Network of Quitlines	www.naquitline.org	1-800-QUIT-NOW

Table 20.13 Paraneoplastic Syndromes with Neuropsychiatric Symptoms

Syndrome	Features	Treatment
SIADH	• Anorexia, Nausea, Vomiting in early stages • Confusion, Convulsions, Coma in late stages • Cerebral edema causes irritability, personality changes, seizures, respiratory arrest	• Tumor treatment/ chemotherapy • Fluid restriction • Hypertonic saline in extreme cases
Hypercalcemia	• Anorexia, Nausea, Vomiting, Constipation, Lethargy • Polyuria, Polydipsia, Dehydration	• Tumor treatment • Reduction of dietary intake • Bisphosphonates • Hydration promoting calciuresis
Lambert-Eaton Myasthenic Syndrome (LEMS)	• Hip girdle muscular weakness initially • Weakness progresses to limbs • Weakness worsens with activity • Electromyography aids diagnosis	• Tumor Treatment • Steroids • Intravenous Immunoglobulin • Plasma Exchange
Limbic Encephalitis	• May predate discovery of malignancy • Rapidly progressive memory problems, new onset psychiatric symptoms • Can include seizures • MRI may show limbic enhancement • Antibody testing available for Anti-Hu, Ma, NMDAR	• Tumor treatment may help • Typically grave prognosis • Supportive measures

Table 20.13 (Continued)

Syndrome	Features	Treatment
Polyneuropathy	• Symmetric distal limb sensorimotor deficits • Subacute type loses of position/vibration sense then pain/temperature sensation • Anti CV2/CRMP5 antibodies may be found	• Tumor treatment may help chronic type • Subacute type is less responsive to treatment, may develop before tumor discovery
Opsoclonus-Myoclonus	• Constant irregular saccades accompanied by truncal ataxia • Adults experience truncal ataxia, gait problems, falls • Confusion may be present • Cerebellar or brainstem signs may occur	• Tumor treatment • Anecdotal evidence for corticosteroids, intravenous immunoglobulin, cyclophosphamide, clonazepam

Adapted from Heinemann S, Zabel P, Hauber H-P. Paraneoplastic syndromes in lung cancer. *Cancer Therapy.* 2008;6:687–98.

References

1. Hutchins LF, Unger JM, Crowley JJ, Coltman CA, Jr., Albain KS. Underrepresentation of patients 65 years of age or older in cancer-treatment trials. *N Engl J Med.* 1999;341(27):2061–2067. doi: 10.1056/NEJM199912303412706

2. Owonikoko TK, Ragin CC, Belani CP, et al. Lung cancer in elderly patients: an analysis of the surveillance, epidemiology, and end results database. *J Clin Oncol.* 2007;25(35):5570–5577. doi: 10.1200/JCO.2007.12.5435

3. American Cancer Society. *Cancer Facts & Figures 2012.* Atlanta, GA: Author; 2012.

4. Kurtz ME, Kurtz JC, Stommel M, Given CW, Given B. Predictors of depressive symptomatology of geriatric patients with lung cancer-a longitudinal analysis. *Psychooncol.* 2002;11(1):12–22.

5. Graves KD, Arnold SM, Love CL, Kirsh KL, Moore PG, Passik SD. Distress screening in a multidisciplinary lung cancer clinic: prevalence and predictors of clinically significant distress. *Lung Cancer.* 2007;55(2):215–224. doi: 10.1016/j.lungcan.2006.10.001

6. Temel ST GJ, Muzikansky A, Gallagher ER, et al. Early palliative care for patients with metastatic non-small-cell lung cancer. *New Eng J Med.* 2010;363:733–742. doi: 10.1056/NEJMoa1000678

7. Gift AG, Jablonski A, Stommel M, Given CW. Symptom clusters in elderly patients with lung cancer. *Oncol Nurs Forum.* 2004;31(2):202–212. doi: 10.1188/04.ONF.202-212. PubMed PMID: 15017438

8. Steward DJ. Lung cancer: prevention, management, and emerging therapies. *Curr Clin Oncol.* 2010:483–502. doi: 10.1007/978-1-60761-524-8

9. Brintzenhofe-Szoc KM. Mixed anxiety/depression symptoms in a large cancer cohort: prevalence by cancer type. *Psychosomat.* 2009;50(4):383–391. doi: 10.1176/appi.psy.50.4.383

10. Bausewein C BS, Gysels M, Higginson I. Non-pharmacological interventions for breathlessness in advanced stages of malignant and non-malignant disease Cochrane Database Syst Rev. 2008(2). doi: 10.1002/14651858. CD005623.pub2

11. Krishnan P, Hawranik P. Diagnosis and management of geriatric insomnia: a guide for nurse practitioners. *J Am Acad Nurse Practition.* 2008;20(12):590–599. doi: 10.1111/j.1745-7599.2008.00366.x. PubMed PMID: 19120590

12. Hopwood P, Stephens RJ. Depression in patients with lung cancer: prevalence and risk factors derived from quality-of-life data. *J Clin Oncol.* 2000;18(4):893–903.

13. Endicott J. Measurement of depression in patients with cancer. *Cancer.* 1984;53(Suppl 10):2243–2249.

14. Walker J, Sawhney A, Hansen CH, Treatment of depression in people with lung cancer: a systematic review. *Lung Cancer.* 2013;79(1):46–53. doi: 10.1016/j.lungcan.2012.09.014. PubMed PMID: 23102652

15. Parsons A, Daley A, Begh R, Aveyard P. Influence of smoking cessation after diagnosis of early stage lung cancer on prognosis: systematic review of observational studies with meta-analysis. BMJ. 2010;340:b5569. doi: 10.1136/bmj.b5569

16. Agency for Healthcare Research and Quality. *Treating Tobacco Use and Dependence.* Rockville, MD: Author; 2013. http://www.ahrq.gov/ professionals/clinicians-providers/guidelines-recommendations/tobacco/ clinicians/update/index.html

17. Heinemann S, Zabel P, Hauber H-P. Paraneoplastic syndromes in lung cancer. *Cancer Therapy.* 2008;6:687–698.

Chapter 21

Colorectal Cancer

Kimberley Miller

Introduction

Colon cancer, the fourth most commonly diagnosed cancer in the United States, is frequently a condition of the older person, with a median age of onset of 69, and is the second leading cause of cancer deaths, with a median age of death of 74.[1] As 65 percent of patients with colorectal cancer (CRC) survive at least 5 years, strategies related to promoting and improving psychosocial adjustment and health-related quality of life become paramount considerations in providing ongoing medical and psychosocial care to this population.

Tables 21.1–21.3 review the unique challenges patients and families face at different points throughout the CRC illness experience (from diagnosis, through treatment, and into survivorship), and possible strategies/responses that may assist the medical teams in their clinical encounters. A review of psychosocial issues related to recurrence, treatment failure, transition to palliative care, and end of life is not provided here, given universal challenges faced by all elderly cancer patients during these points in illness trajectory. They are discussed in Chapter 14. Patients with terminal CRC may suffer from pain related to bowel obstruction, profound fatigue, weakness and/or delirium from widely metastatic liver involvement, and thus managing these symptoms remains of upmost importance in minimizing and alleviating distress in the advanced CRC setting.

Elderly CRC patients may be at greatest risk of developing anxiety and depression soon after diagnosis,[2] but should continue to be assessed, when clinically indicated. Psychosocial screening instruments are discussed in Chapter 4. Predictors of the development of depressive symptoms over time have been found to include higher cancer-related symptoms, limitations in physical and social functioning (highlighting the need for individualized symptom management and assisting patients to mobilize social support), medical comorbidity, female gender, and African American race.[2]

Approximately 40 percent of patients present with Stage I disease and have a 90 percent chance of surviving 5 years or longer, whereas those who present with advanced disease have a 12.5 percent chance of surviving beyond 5 years,[1] emphasizing the need to assess the individual priorities, as well as the estimated lifespan, of each patient, when guiding them through

Table 21.1 Adjusting to Diagnosis

Patient Challenge	Strategy/Response by Medical Team
Difficulty making treatment decision	• Educate patient and family about goals of treatment (e.g. to prolong life, maintain function and independence, palliate symptoms) and potential treatment responses/toxicities; help them to weigh toxicity risk, QOL (e.g., coping with stoma/ostomy) and survival advantage; explore fear, uncertainty about future.
	• Use tools to guide treatment decisions, including geriatric assessment scores, comorbidity indices, frailty indices, scores for predicting toxicity from chemotherapy, prognostic indices for survival.[3]
	• Educate patients and families through larger teaching sessions about various treatments (e.g., surgery, including ostomy/stoma; chemotherapy; radiation).
	• Use tumor boards with multidisciplinary input, including geriatrician, if available.
Anxiety related to treatment response and tolerability	• Inform patient and family of surveillance plan (follow up appointments, imaging/colonoscopies/tumor markers), expected toxicities & team response, available resources.
	• If curative intent, encourage "eye on the prize" psychology; "short term pain for long-term gain", help them to consider how they might reward themselves at end of treatment.
	• If treatment more palliative in nature, validate and explore fears about future dependency, suffering, dying, separation from family refer to palliative care, begin discussions re: goals of care, discuss "hoping for the best, preparing for the worst" approach.
Guilt re: lack/delay of screening	• Nonjudgmentally explore motivation for avoidance (e.g., often involves fear of procedure, receiving bad news), and facilitate expression of emotions including guilt, disappointment, fear, and anger.
	• If family history present, explore their experience of family member's CRC, and relationship to their own (lack/delay of) screening and assumptions about their own future.
	• Explore fear of disclosing to family members if genetically increased risk of CRC present.
	• Focus them on present treatment and making best decisions for themselves moving forward.
Adjustment in Roles/ Relationships	• Empathically explore anticipated challenges of the change in their role in context of multiple other losses with age, including social (e.g., loss of family members, friends, financial (e.g., fixed income) and health (e.g., medical comorbidities); emphasize underlying patient strengths in coping with current transition, relate it to how they have positively coped through previous transitions.
	• Provide referral for financial resources re: transportation (e.g., daily radiation) and housing (e.g. patients who do not reside in the area where treatment offered).
	• Refer to support groups, volunteer patients (including those with ostomy), stoma nurse.

Table 21.2 Adjusting to Treatment

Patient Challenge	Strategy/Response by Medical Team
Coping with toxicities	• In metastatic patients, stop-and-go or maintenance monotherapy strategies during combination therapy may help minimize toxicity and risk of feeling cancer not being treated.
	• Hematological toxicities and mucositis may be more common with chemotherapy in elderly; higher rates of toxicities seen with bevacizumab, mainly thromboembolic events, so education and monitoring/preparation for these risks advised.[4]
	• If mucositis develops, may need to switch oral medications to alternate route temporarily (e.g., re: psychotropic medications: consider mirtazapine Rapid Dissolve (RD), olanzapine zydis, risperidone m-tab, escitalopram meltz, lorazepam sublingual (SL)/intravenous (IV), haloperidol IV).
	• Educate re: Oxaliplatin neuropathy may involve paresthesia, hypoesthesia, and changes in proprioception that can affect fine motor coordination (e.g. writing, buttoning, picking up small objects) as well as gait abnormalities.[5]
Adjustment to Stoma/Ostomy	• Involve enterostomy nurse and/or volunteer patient (ideally preoperatively) to provide education on wound and ostomy care, strategies to deal with incontinence/flatulence (e.g., special bags, simethicone), leakage, odor and noise, body image (e.g., ways to conceal bag), empowering self-care.
	• Address misconceptions and assumptions about living with ostomy/stoma.
	• Address financial resources in paying for equipment.
	• Ask about impact on sexual functioning, assess need for couple's counselling.
	• Involve dietician.

the treatment decision process. Those with more advanced disease will have different psychosocial needs than those facing earlier stage disease, although there will clearly be some overlap in the challenges faced, as reflected Tables 21.1–21.3.

Chronological age has not been found to be a valid criterion on which to base treatment decision, although is often a strong factor in withholding CRC treatment in elderly patients, especially chemotherapy. Rather than relying solely on age, a comprehensive geriatric assessment, including assessment of factors including functional status, nutrition, cognition, and socioeconomic and emotional status, is suggested.[3] Tables 21.1 and 21.2 review challenges related to adjusting to diagnosis and treatment; Table 21.3 highlights problems faced by CRC survivors. An in-depth discussion on the use of psychopharmacological interventions is beyond the scope of this chapter; management of psychiatric disorders can be found in Chapter 7. However, unique considerations when prescribing psychotropic medications in colorectal cancer patients include: some selective serotonin reuptake inhibitors (e.g., escitalopram, citalopram, sertraline,) may contribute to slighter looser stool; tricyclic antidepressants, serotonin norepinephrine reuptake inhibitors (e.g., duloxetine, venlafaxine), mirtazapine, and bupropion are more constipating; and mirtazapine and olanzapine have been shown to be useful for management of nausea.

Table 21.3 Adjusting to Survivorship

Patient Challenge	Strategy/Response by Medical Team
Dealing with ongoing GI symptoms (e.g., diarrhea, stool leakage, incontinence)	• Recommend antidiarrheal medications, e.g., loperamide, lomotil. • Educate re: need for regular irrigation of ostomy. • Bowel training regimen.
Sexual functioning	• Enquire about sexual activity predating CRC treatment, and provide education re: risk of injury to pelvic nerves during surgery and damage from radiation (RT); assess for any changes in sexual functioning/activity during and after treatment. In women, RT can cause vaginal atrophy, fibrosis, adhesions and shortening of vagina; treatment may require vaginal dilators, lubrication, recommendations of nonintercourse sexual activities. In men, ED is a common (especially when comorbidity present, e.g., diabetes) complication of rectal surgery and RT, and can be treated with ED medications (e.g., sildenafil). • Manage previously mentioned GI symptoms optimally to minimize role of social embarrassment contributing to sexual dysfunction/avoidance of sexual activity. • Discuss impact SD having on couple and refer to sexual rehabilitation services, couples counseling, if available.

References

1. Howlader N, Noone AM, Krapcho M, et al., eds. *SEER Cancer Statistics Review, 1975–2011*. Bethesda, MD: National Cancer Institute; 2013. http://seer.cancer.gov/csr/1975_2011/, based on November 20132 SEER data submission, posted to the SEER web site, April 2014.

2. Kurtz ME, Kurtz JC, Stommel M, Given CW, Given B. Predictors of depressive symptomatology of geriatric patients with colorectal cancer. *Support Cancer Care* 2002;10:494–501.

3. Leo S, Accetura C, Gnoni A, et al. Systemic treatment of gastrointestinal cancer in elderly patients. *J Gastrointest Canc* 2013;44:22–32.

4. Kozloff MF, Berlin J, Flynn PJ, et al. Clinical outcomes in elderly patients with metastatic colorectal cancer receiving bevacizumab and chemotherapy: results from the BRiTE observational cohort study. *Oncology* 2010;78:329–339.

5. Holt PR, Kozuch P, Mewar S. Clon cancer and the elderly: from screening to treatment in management of GI disease in the elderly. *Best Pract Res & Clin Gastroenterol.* 2009;23:889–907.

Chapter 22

Leukemia and Lymphoma

Tomer T. Levin

Hematological malignancies are largely diseases of the elderly and their incidence increases with age as illustrated in Table 22.1. The intersection of aging and these malignancies creates unique psychosocial challenges, which are considered in this chapter.

Communication

The terms leukemia and lymphoma can be both frightening and poorly understood by patients and families. It is helpful to teach them the specific name of their hematological malignancy, for example, "You have a slow growing cancer of your white blood cells called chronic lymphocytic leukemia or CLL. Let me write this down and tell you more about what this means..." This educational process helps to minimize emotional catastrophizing and misperceptions about what a "blood cancer" means.

- Patients should be taught the acronyms and names of the treatments (e.g., R-CHOP) to avoid misperceptions that "chemo" refers to a toxic chemical.
- Patients with hematological malignancies often feel marginalized because they have no obvious treatment deformity such as is seen in breast or colon cancer; family and friends may not appreciate the gravity of their illness. Clinicians will need to educate patients about their illness and patients, in turn can educate their families and friends.
- Empathically address the emotional impact of a leukemia or lymphoma diagnosis on the patient and family with statements such as, "I know this was unexpected..." or "I appreciate how difficult it must be to hear that you have CLL..."
- When speaking to a geriatric patient and an accompanying third person, such as a family member, friend, or carer, beware of marginalizing the patient by mainly addressing the third person. Decisions should be based on the principles of shared decision making, to the greatest degree that this is possible, so as to respect the patient's autonomy.

Table 22.1 Median Age of Diagnosis of Hematological Malignancies	
Hematological Malignancy	**Median Age of Diagnosis (Years)**
Chronic Myeloid Leukemia	67
Chronic Lymphocytic Leukemia	72
Hairy cell leukemia	50 (bimodal: peaks at 40 & 80)
Polycythemia Vera	60–66
Essential thrombocythemia	60
Primary myelofibrosis	60
Acute lymphocytic leukemia	13 (bimodal: peaks childhood & 70–90)
Acute myeloid leukemia	67 (incidence rises consistently with age)
Non-Hodgkin lymphoma	66

Adapted from Wiernik PH, Goldman JM, Dutcher JP, Kyle RA. *Neoplastic Diseases of the Blood*. 5th ed. New York, NY: Springer; 2013.

Watch and Wait

Chronic lymphocytic leukemia and indolent lymphomas are often treated with watch and wait monitoring, the standard of care for many, early-stage, slow-growing lymphomas. Watching and waiting, however, in a technological world that expects instant gratification can be anxiety provoking.

- Rates of anxiety and depression are not higher in watch and wait versus actively treated or later stage disease. Older patients are not more vulnerable to watch and wait anxiety, in fact anxiety tends to decrease with age.[2]
- Anxiety and depression should be assessed and treated appropriately, usually with cognitive therapy, and/or SSRI plus benzodiazepine, or benzodiazepine alone.

Pain and Depression

With bone involvement, multiple myeloma is particularly debilitating in the elderly.

- Remember: acute pain causes anxiety; chronic pain causes depression.
- SNRIs target such as venlafaxine and duloxetine target both serotonergic and noradrenergic pathways and have a theoretical advantage over SSRIs such as citalopram, because serotonergic pathways are not involved in pain modulation.
- Venlafaxine dose should be decreased in renal failure. Less common side effects include hyponatremia and hypertension in doses above 150mg/day. Less serious side effects include a dry mouth, insomnia, and nausea. Duloxetine should not be given to patients with liver failure or those who abuse alcohol or are dependent upon it and it can also cause usually reversible transaminitis. Postural hypotension can be problematic especially if the patient is already taking antihypertensive

medications. When stopping both of these medications, a taper will reduce the chance of serotonin withdrawal syndrome. The risk of increased hemorrhage, especially gastrointestinal bleeding is of concern in the elderly; increased vigilance should be applied to patients already taking anticoagulants or aspirin.

- SSRIs and SNRIs are effective for anxiety and depression in the elderly but the long course of treatment, 6–12 months and often longer may be burdensome and expensive.
- Opioids and benzodiazepines increase the risk for delirium in the elderly.

Caregiver Burnout

Caregiver burnout—physical and emotional exhaustion, often accompanied by financial stress—is common. On average, 20.4 hours/week are spent by a caregiver, which is disruptive to maintaining a work-life balance. The use of physiological rather than absolute age, and gentler, better-tolerated treatments such as nonablative, T-cell depleted allogeneic transplants, and outpatient autologous stem cell transplants, all mean that elderly leukemia and lymphoma patients are treated more aggressively and for longer. Pneumonia, a common complication of treatments, was once known colloquially as the old man's friend, but now is treated in intensive care settings, creating a new category of frailty, the chronic critically ill. All these factors may add to caregiver burden, and this is more pronounced when the primary caregiver is also elderly. The management of caregiver burnout is multifactorial and is addressed using all the resources of the multidisciplinary team, the patient's family and community, and with the assistance of respite care where available.

Screening

Before starting an arduous treatment such as stem cell transplantation, psychosocial screening can identify those at greater risk to facilitate earlier or prophylactic treatment. Screen for:

- Current depression and anxiety levels. Validated instruments such as the Geriatric Depression Scale, Patient Health Questionnaire-9 and the Generalized Anxiety Disorder Questionnaire are freely available online, but patients with cognitive or visual impairment may be better served by simple one-line screeners such as asking, "Are you depressed?"
- Past history of depression and anxiety disorders, bipolar disorder or postnatal depression, and prior psychiatric treatment.
- Family history of psychiatric problems such as bipolar disorder.
- Alcohol and substance abuse, past and current.
- Prior episodes of delirium. This is helpful in developing strategies to reduce the likelihood of delirium developing in high-risk situations such as pending elective surgery.

- Cognitive dysfunction, using instruments such as the Mini Mental Examination, Draw a Clock, and the Montreal Cognitive Assessment.

Prophylactic antidepressants can be helpful for patients with a past history of depression or anxiety or where it seems likely that arduous treatments such as stem cell transplantation might precipitate depression, but there is no data supporting the notion that global prophylaxis with antidepressants improves outcomes.

Cognitive Impairment

Elderly patients are often wary of treatments that might cause neurocognitive damage and worsen their memory. Indeed, even a small drop in cognitive function can be disastrous for someone with little reserve. Baseline cognitive screening or comprehensive psychological testing can be helpful to quantify the deficit. Neuroimaging is helpful to diagnosis stroke, metastases, leptomeningeal disease, normal pressure hydrocephalus, dementia, and other neurological conditions. An electroencephalogram is occasionally helpful when a seizure is present or to substantiate the diagnosis of delirium where a pattern of low-frequency, generalized slowing is seen. Other points to note are that:

- **High dose steroids** pose a greater risk of steroid neuropsychiatric toxicity in the elderly. Many leukemia and lymphoma treatment regimens include steroids, often at high doses; clinicians should be vigilant for mood changes that can manifest as anxiety, depression, hypomania or full-blown mania and occasionally confusion. Anecdotal evidence points to the utility of a low-dose antipsychotic mood stabilizer such olanzapine 2.5 mg per day for hypomanic symptoms and also anxiety and insomnia.

- **Informed consent with comorbid dementia and a treatable hematological malignancy.** Dementia creates an ethical issue in elderly patients with comorbid dementia and a treatable, often curable hematological illness, such as Non-Hodgkin's Lymphoma. If patients lack capacity to make medical decisions, who should weigh up the risks and benefits of cancer treatments on their behalf? These treatments carry a considerable burden of suffering, and risk of death, albeit at the benefit of extending life. The extension of life when a person has dementia needs to be tailored to their and their family's outlook on life. Such issues should be actively debated among clinicians and families, and often both parties benefit from an expert ethics consultation.

- **Delirium:** this is seen in up to 50 percent of hospitalized patients and the primary treatment is to remove the underlying trigger, which is not uncommonly a drug toxicity, a drug interaction or other reversible medical factors such as infection, stroke, seizures, electrolyte abnormalities, cardiac ischemia or substance withdrawal. Using antipsychotics such as low dose, intravenous haloperidol may reduce the duration of the confusion but non-drug treatments that aim to improve sleep quality, reassure patients, and help them to process their environment such as hanging family photos in the hospital room, are all useful. Forty percent of patients may suffer from incomplete resolution of the delirium. Falls risk is greatly increased in this subgroup.

Fatigue

Fatigue is an important symptom to address as it is seen frequently in this population. After treatment of all reversible factors contributing toward fatigue, for example, anemia, a stimulant such as low dose methylphenidate (5–20 mg at breakfast and lunch, as needed) is often helpful. Stimulants must be used with care in the elderly with preexisting cardiac disease, and these patients must be carefully monitored for tachycardia, angina, and arrhythmias. Low impact exercise also has documented positive effects on chronic fatigue in cancer patients.

Prognosis

Prognosis is an issue that frustrates elderly patients who are both grasping for hope and practically planning for their futures.

- Discuss prognosis using the best, most likely, and worst-case scenarios. Median survival data can be mapped onto this—the most likely outcome is half to double the median survival, the best case 4–6 times the median, and the worst case about one-sixth of the median.[3]
- When discussing prognosis, it is essential to outline the action plan for the worst-case scenario. This reassures patients and their families that they will not be abandoned, even when treatment seems futile and death is approaching.

Palliative Care

The palliative trajectory in hematological malignancies is not as predictable as compared with solid tumors. Patients who are critically ill frequently improve and are cured, whereas others die. One in five Americans die in intensive care units, and this is an undesirable palliative-care outcome because it makes a "good death" more elusive.

- Introduce the notion of palliative care early and educate patients and families about resources.
- Utilize a palliative-care approach to symptom relief, quality of life, and planning for death, in tandem to life-extending treatments, and not serially as a default after treatment failure.
- Tailor end-of-life care to patients' values and expectations.
- Use the directive term *Allow Natural Death* rather than *Do Not Resuscitate*, because this links into the goals of care discussion in a more fluid manner.

References

1. Wiernik PH, Goldman JM, Dutcher JP, Kyle RA. *Neoplastic Diseases of the Blood*. 5th ed. New York, NY: Springer; 2013.

2. Levin TT, Li Y, Riskind J, Rai K. Depression, anxiety and quality of life in a chronic lymphocytic leukemia cohort. *Gen Hosp Psychiat*. 2007;29:251–256.

3. Kiely BE, Tattersall MH, Stockler MR. Certain death in uncertain time: informing hope by quantifying a best case scenario. *J Clin Oncol*. 2010;28:2802–2804.

Appendix

National Resources

Anne Martin

Resources for Elderly Cancer Patients

Listed below are some national resources that may provide assistance to older oncology patients and their families. Please consult state and city websites for resources in your local area.

Asian American Resources

Asian American Cancer Support
www.aacsn.org/helpfulresources.html

American Cancer Society Asian Initiatives
www.cancer.org/InYourArea/asian-initiatives

Caregiver Services

Alzheimer's Association
www.alz.org

National Family Caregivers Association
www.thefamilycaregiver.org

Family Caregiver Alliance: National Center on Caregiving
www.caregiver.org

Clinical Trials

Lazerax Cancer Foundation
www.lazerax.org

Education and Support

American Cancer Society
www.cancer.org

Cancer Care, Inc.
www.cancercare.org

Cancer Support Community
www.csc.org.

Patient Resource Cancer Guide
www.patientresource.net

Elder Abuse

National Center on Elder Abuse
http://www.ncea.aoa.gov/Stop_Abuse/GetHelp/State/index.aspx

Food Service Programs

Meals-on-Wheels Association of America
http://www.mowaa.org/page.aspx?pid=253

Financial Assistance

Patient Advocate Foundation
http://www.patientadvocate.org/

American Cancer Society
www.cancer.org/

Cancer Care, Inc.
www.cancercare.org

The Health Well Foundation
www.healthwellfoundation.org

Government Resources

Social Security Administration
http://www.ssa.gov

Administration on Aging
www.aoa.gov

National Cancer Institute
www.cancer.gov

Homecare

Case Manager's Resource Guide Online
http://www.cmrg.com.

National Association for Homecare and Hospice
http://www.nahcagencylocator.com

Hospice

Hospice Association of America
http://www.nahc.org/haa

Hospice Education Institute
http://www.hospiceworld.org/

National Hospice & Palliative Care Organization
www.nhpco.org

Housing

SeniorHousingNet
www.seniorhousing.net/seniors

Nursing Home Compare
http://www.medicare.gov/NHcompare/home.asp

Alternatives for Seniors
http://www.alternativesforseniors.com

Legal Assistance

National Academy of Elder Law Attorneys
www.naela.org

U.S. Citizenship and Immigration Services
www.uscis.gov

The Medicare Rights Center
www.medicarerights.org

LGBT Resources

Services & Advocacy for GLBT Elders (SAGE)
http://www.sageusa.org/index.cfm

National LGBT Cancer Network
info@cancer-network.org

Mental Health

American Psychosocial Oncology Society
http://www.apos-society.org/survivors/helpline/helpline.aspx

American Association of Geriatric Psychiatry
www.aagpgpa.org

American Delirium Society
www.americandeliriumsociety.org

American Geriatrics Society
www.americangeriatrics.org

Association of Oncology Social Workers
www.aosw.org

Geriatric Mental Health Association
www.gmhfonline.org/gmhf/find.asp

International Psychosocial Oncology Society
www.ipos-society.org

Mental Health America
http://www.mentalhealthamerica.net

Veterans and Military Health
www.nlm.nih.gov/medlineplus/veteransandmilitaryhealth.html

Prescription Medication

Extra Help
http://www.ssa.gov/prescriptionhelp/index.htm

Free Medicine Bureau of Prescription Help
www.freemedicine.com

NeedyMeds
www.needymeds.com

Patient Advocate Foundation
www.patientadvocate.org

Partnership for Prescription Assistance
https://www.pparx.org/Intro.php

Rx Savings Plus
www.Rxsavingsplus.com

Sun Patient Prescription Card
http://sunassociation.org/index.php

Spanish Resources

American Cancer Society
http://www.cancer.org/Espanol/index

Cancer Care
http://www.cancercare.org/espanol

National Cancer Institute
http://www.cancer.gov/espanol

Cancer.Net
cancer.net/espanol

Substance Abuse

Alcoholics Anonymous
www.aa.org

Al-Anon Family Groups
http://www.al-anon.alateen.org

American Addiction Centers
americanaddictioncenters.com

American Society of Addiction Medicine (ASAM)
http://www.asam.org

Survivorship

National Coalition for Cancer Survivorship
http://www.canceradvocacy.org

National Cancer Institute: Office of Cancer Survivorship
http://dccps.nci.nih.gov/ocs/office-survivorship.html

LIVESTRONG
www.livestrong.org

Transportation

Corporate Angels Network
www.corpangelnetwork.org

Air Charity Network
www.aircharitynetwork.org

Mercy Medical Airlift
mercymedical.org

Volunteer/Paid Opportunities

Senior Corps
http://www.seniorcorps.org/

Encore
http://www.encore.org/about

AARP Experience Corps
www.americorps.gov

Index